D0961141

SUPER
POTENCY
AT ANY AGE

SUPER
POTENCY
AT ANY AGE

EDWIN FLATTO, M.D.

Instant Improvement, Inc.

Instant Improvement, Inc.
210 East 86th Street
New York, New York 10028

Library of Congress Cataloging-in-Publication Data

Flatto, Edwin.
    Super potency at any age / Edwin Flatto.
        p.   cm.
    Includes bibliographical references and index.
    ISBN 0-941683-09-5
    1. Impotence—Prevention. 2. Impotence—Exercise therapy.
3. Impotence—Diet Therapy. I. Title.
RC889.F53   1991
616.6'9205—dc20   91-73635

Important

You will find Dr. Flatto's advice extremely valuable in following your personal physician's recommendations. The information provided is for your better health. However, any decision you make involving the treatment of an illness should include your family doctor. Naturally, since individual metabolisms vary, not everyone can experience identical or optimum results. Before beginning any program of exercise, please consult your physician.

Acknowledgements

First, I want to express my gratitude to my dear friend and publisher, Gene Schwartz.

A special thanks to Frank Ray Rifkin and Andrew Rifkin, editors and publishers of *Nutrition Health Review* and *Consumers Medical Journal* for permission to use some of the questions and answers from my medical column which appears in their publications.

To all my patients and dear friends whose life experiences have been enriched through principles and techniques included in this book. To all of you I say, "Thank You." May God grant you strength to continue your good work for many more years to come.

There is a destiny that makes us brothers,
None goes his way alone.
All that we send into the lives of others
Comes back into our own.

Author unknown

Contents

Introduction

AS A PRACTICING INTERNIST, I AM CONSTANTLY beleaguered by maturing men who complain, frequently too late, of waning sexual powers and urinary function. It is therefore of utmost interest to me to have met a doctor who seems to have avoided what others have accepted as a necessary concomitant of aging.

Extensive interview and examination have impressed me with the author's remarkable vitality, youthfulness and knowledge of genito-urinary function.

In these modern times with the accent on youthfulness, vigor and machismo, that poor soul who cannot perform lustily is left alone with his sad complexes or must resort to mutilating surgery, dangerous injections, or tablets with treacherous side effects. Is he not infinitely better off with a program of sensible diet, exercise, and modification of his behavior? Having witnessed disastrous failure and having struggled to undo these side effects, I feel that I'm eminently qualified to answer in the affirmative. And as a maturing male, I have a personal interest in this subject.

All doctors wish to be held as gods to their patients, and conversely all patients wish to be the recipient of medical magic and skill. Thus, if a program to avoid major emotional and physical distress is available, it behooves both doctor and patient to embrace it enthusiastically. However, if there were even one small element that might be unhealthy, it should be candidly exposed and discarded.

Dr. Flatto's principles, self-applied with such great success, can be scrutinized in this respect. It is inconceivable to me that harm could result from following his recommendations. There is nothing bizarre, unsupported by medical evidence, or dangerous in the diet and exercises he recommends. He may very well make you the envy of your peers.

The world has become increasingly health-conscious. Greater emphasis is placed on preventive medicine, making this book extremely timely. It is imperative that our eating and exercise habits require marked and prompt change if we are to avoid those degenerative diseases associated with aging.

It seems somewhat unscientific to advocate common sense when people are much more impressed with technology, computers, and machinery. There is a frightening inclination to disregard history and experience. Medicine, not being an exact science, cannot afford this luxury!

Robert Rosenblum, M.D.

Preface

I WROTE THIS BOOK PRIMARILY TO HELP MEN achieve more meaningful, happier, healthier and fulfilling lives. But I hope women will read it too. Every woman has men who are deeply involved in her life: father, brother, husband, lover, son, etc., whose sexual health and virility are important factors in their happiness and fulfillment.

It should be axiomatic that our Creator endowed every man with the potential ability to perform the sexual act for as long as he lives. And the scientific evidence supports this premise. It is only because man is his own worst enemy that he has deprived himself of his natural heritage. By his own unnatural living habits, man has only deprived himself of a lifetime of sexual fulfillment—and his health and happiness in other areas have suffered as well.

He has brought upon himself degenerative diseases that our Creator never intended for him to endure. Atherosclerosis, heart disease, cancer, constipation, emphysema, arthritis, back-ache, prostate disease and impotence were not part of our Creator's plan for human destiny.

11

There is no disease or death that was ever caused by "old age," per se. There is always a breakdown or toxemic condition of one or more vital organs of the body. It is man's unnatural living habits that cause delayed elimination, toxic buildup, and, finally, breakdown.

There is no organ in man's body that was not given a potential useful life of over a hundred years, and that applies to man's sex organs too. The French scientist, Alexis Carrel, demonstrated that a chicken heart can be kept alive indefinitely if the toxins are removed from the blood that feeds it. I believe the same applies to the human heart.

If man ate the food nature equipped him to eat, exercised his body the way nature intended, and eliminated all toxic habits that have become part of our "civilization," man could live far beyond what is considered "old age" and have perfect health.

According to the Bible, "And all the days that Adam lived, were nine hundred and thirty years. And he begat sons and daughters. And Seth lived after he begat Enos eight hundred and seven years and begat sons and daughters. And Enos lived after he begat Cainan, eight hundred and fifteen years and begat sons and daughters. And Cainan lived seventy years and begat Mahalaleel; and Cainan lived after he begat Mahalaleel eight hundred and forty years and begat sons and daughters. And all the days of Cainan were nine hundred and ten years." Genesis, Chapter 5.

I could go on quoting Genesis, which chronicles the beginnings of recorded history, to show that ancient man lived over eight hundred years and "begat sons and daughters until his death." But some people find it hard to believe that man, at eight hundred years of age, was still sexually active.

In those days, man breathed pure air, drank unpolluted water, and didn't smoke. His food supply was eaten the way Nature intended: uncontaminated, uncooked, organically grown fresh fruits and vegetables. Drugs, either prescription or over-the-counter, were unknown to him. There were no automobiles or buses in those days, so man had to walk, climb, or run whenever he wanted to go somewhere. I believe that this pristine state of affairs enabled these giants of men to live in such perfect health and to still be potent at an advanced age.

I have not written this book to help people live to a ripe old age spent in pain, disease, in a hospital bed or in some other miserable existence. I would not want to live to an old age in such a state, and I believe there aren't many others who would.

Fortunately, however, it is possible to lead a healthful and vigorous life up to and beyond the point which is normally regarded as "old age." We shall, of course, grow old in years, but if we live in harmony with nature's laws, we need not grow old in mind or heart, nor need we lose our physical energy, our alertness and suppleness of body and mind long before the expiration of our allotted time. While growing old in years, we can grow younger and more robust as far as our intellectual, emotional, and moral qualities are concerned.

In nature, each species of animal appears to have a certain age limit; when this limit is reached, the animal declines rapidly and dies. It does not spend a third of its normal lifetime getting old and dying, as does the average human being. On the contrary, the animal retains its full vigor and beauty of form almost to the very end of its life span.

Just as there are definite laws that govern the universe and guide the moon and stars in their precise path in the heavens, so there are precise natural laws that govern our bodies. And it is only through obedience to these laws that our destiny of vigorous, vital health and potency at any age can be achieved.

Chapter 1

Lifelong Potency: Every Man's Birthright

S OME PEOPLE ACCEPT AS A MAXIM THAT SEX
is only for the young and we must give it up as we
age. There are a number of reasons why the physical ability to
perform sex decreases with age and almost all of them can be
avoided or reversed. In this book I will explain what factors
decrease potency, which ones increase your ability to perform,
and how proper diet and exercise can help you attain a lifetime
of sexual fulfillment.

Erection: Normal Function

In the penis there are two long, thin chambers filled with
spongy tissue called the corpora cavernosa. They are normally
empty and relatively dry. An erection is brought about by
blood that rushes in from the penile arteries, thereby engorging
the erectile tissue and causing the penis to expand. As arterial
inflow increases and venous outflow decreases, the penis at first
becomes enlarged, and then fully rigid. This is brought about
by reflex action stimulated by the brain through psychic
stimulation and communicated through the central nervous
system, or through tactile stimulation of sensory nerve endings
of erogenous zones. Blood is trapped in the penile chambers by
valves. Valves are also controlled by reflex action, not voluntary
control (this is why one cannot simply will an erection).
Testosterone, secreted by the Leydig cells of the penis, facilitates
penile erection through an unknown mechanism. Any block-

age of the penile arteries and/or their contributory blood vessels will prevent or impede an erection; normal sexual functioning depends on intact circulatory, neural, and hormonal systems.[1,2]

Effects of Aging on Sexual Function

The ability to have erections and ejaculations is not lost with aging. Physical problems that occur are usually treatable and may be avoided altogether through proper diet and exercise. Sexual desire does not wane with aging, even in men suffering from erectile dysfunction. It usually takes a longer time and more direct stimulation to get an erection. Frequently the time before an erection can occur again is longer. The number of spontaneous erections also are fewer. Sperm production generally ends in the seventies, although there are men who remain fertile into their nineties. These are all completely normal changes and do not necessarily mean a decline in potency.[3]

These "effects" of aging may be no more than an indication of the effects of wrong diet, lack of proper exercise, and disease in the male population. With right nutrition and exercises, I believe that full sexual potency can continue throughout life.

Impotency

Sexual problems have been recorded throughout history. Ancient Egyptian papyri gave recipes to cure impotence as early as 431 B.C. Hippocrates thought that impotence could be caused by unattractiveness in women and preoccupation with business. One of the earliest cases of sexual impotency is recorded in the Bible, when King David was forced to relinquish his throne because he was unable to perform. (1 Kings 1:2,4,5)

Although school children's books don't often mention it, another well-documented case of erectile dysfunction involved Louis XVI of France (reign 1774-1792), who at sixteen years of age was married to Marie Antoinette, age fifteen. According to the medical literature, for the first seven years of their marriage, the young monarch was totally impotent and therefore unable to consummate the marriage. Various letters and medical dispatches about the king's problem circulated among diplomatic and medical circles, and the public was undoubtedly aware of the royal problem. Finally, physicians determined that the problem was a tight prepuce or foreskin. After excision of the prepuce (circumcision), the problem was corrected, and in 1785 the couple had a son, Louis XVII. Their sex lives were apparently happy until the French revolution, when both were guillotined.[4]

What exactly is impotency? It is usually defined as inability of the male organ to become erect and perform the sexual act. Some doctors further define impotency as being either orgasmic or erectile in nature. "Orgasmic impotence would refer to the absence of or difficulty in achieving orgasm as well as the quick achievement of orgasm normally termed premature ejaculation. The most common form of impotence would be erectile impotence—the patient cannot achieve or maintain a satisfactory erection.[5]

Impotence should not be confused with sterility. Impotency is inability of the male organ to become erect. Sterility is inability through organic defect to produce offspring. An impotent man may have sperm that are viable and healthy and therefore are not sterile. A sterile man may sustain an erection and indulge in sexual relations, but the sterile man is like a hunter who only shoots blanks. Neither should impotence be confused with loss of libido, or, simply, lack of interest in sex.

It is estimated that 14% of American men suffer from chronic impotence, a total of 20 million men. At the age of sixty, 25% of men are impotent; at the age of seventy, 60% are no longer able to perform; and by age eighty, 85% are impotent.[6] However, more than 50% of men over the age of eighty report continued interest in sex.[7] Considering there are three women for every man at age eighty, and only one man out of four is still sexually active, it presents a marvelous opportunity for eighty-year-old men still potent!

There are different degrees of impotency: partial or complete, temporary, situational and inconsistent. Potency varies in healthy men from time to time. All men at some time in their lives experience temporary erection problems for various reasons: anxiety, stress, fatigue, fear, and excessive alcohol abuse. Many other factors can cause temporary impotence. The stresses of moving, a job change, financial worries, and just plain fatigue can suppress sexual desires. Sometimes a social problem within the home can interfere with sexual functioning, such as a parent living in the home or small children who wander into the bedroom without warning. Other factors such as a history of sexual abuse or fear of getting herpes or AIDs can cause erectile problems.

The causes of potency problems are numerous. There are physical as well as psychogenic or emotional causes, and impotence may be due to a combination of the two. Until relatively recent times, it was believed that 90% of all male impotency was psychogenic. Sigmund Freud first propounded this theory. For the next fifty years this theory was generally accepted as truth. However, new research using penile Dopplers and other measuring devices have shown that over 50% of all impotence results from physical causes. Treating these patients with psychotherapy is as useless as treating psychological impotence with surgery.

Diet and general health play an important part in determining ability as well as desire to perform the sexual act. For example, the high-fat, low-fiber typical American diet which emphasizes meat, eggs, cheese, fish, as well as alcohol, spicy foods, and salt, may stimulate desire for sex but tends to decrease ability to perform. Nicotine, morphine, and cocaine are all anaphrodisiacs, or sexual depressants. In a recent review of medical literature, over 85% of patients with impotence from occlusion of blood vessels of the penis had histories of high blood pressure, high cholesterol levels, cigarette smoking, or diabetes mellitus.[8]

Sexual potency as well as sperm formation can also be inhibited by some drugs. Alcohol, nicotine (both of these substances are drugs although they are not usually considered as such), barbiturates, antihistamines, antidepressants, heart medications, marijuana and some drugs prescribed for diabetes, stomach ulcers, and high blood pressure have all been reported in medical journals as causing impotence as a side effect. Ionizing radiation (radioactivity and X-ray), prolonged exposure to defective microwave ovens or radar, and exposure to toxic substances with which industrial workers come into prolonged contact can all impair normal sperm formation and potency.

Diseases That Cause Potency Problems

Certain diseases that impede blood circulation by constricting or occluding arteries or by adversely affecting the central nervous system can cause impotence, sterility, or both. One British study of diabetes stated that about 50% of all diabetics complain of impotence. Obesity is known to decrease potency, so that should be a strong incentive to help you stick to a diet. A New York urologist who did a study of 300 cases of impotence reported that 44% had a history of gonorrhea. In the latter stages of syphilis, loss of potency may be one of the early symptoms. Remember, promiscuity increases your risk of contracting life-threatening disease. Nature helps the sexual needy—not the greedy!

Physical causes of impotency:

Atherosclerosis

Hypertension

Diabetes mellitus

Alcohol abuse

Smoking

Drug abuse

Liver or kidney failure

Parkinson's disease

Fractures or surgery in the pelvic area (prostate, bladder, rectum, etc.)

Spinal cord injuries

Multiple sclerosis

Peyronie's disease (curvature of the penis)

Priapism (persistent abnormal penis erection)

Congenital problems of sexual organ development

Congenital hormonal problems

Sickle-cell anemia

Hyper- and hypothyroidism

Aortic aneurysm surgery

Heavy metal poisoning, such as lead

Cancer and radiation treatments

Amyotrophic lateral sclerosis (Lou Gehrig's disease)

Prostate disease

Direct injury to the penis

Leriche's syndrome

References

1.   Brooks, M. *Lifelong Sexual Vigor.* (Garden City, NY: Doubleday, 1981), 11-16.

2.   Mulligan, T., and P. G. Katz. "Erectile Failure in the Aged." *Journal of the American Geriatrics Society.* 36 (1988), 54-62.

3.   Butler, R. N., and M. I. Lewis. *Love and Sex After 60.* (New York: Harper and Row, 1988), 26-27.

4.   Brooks, M. op. cit., 7-8.

5.   Cartmill, R. A. "The Ups and Downs of Impotence." *Australian Family Physician.* 18:3 (Mar 1989), 213.

6.   Masters, W.H., and V. E. Johnson. *Human Sexual Inadequacy.* (London: Churchill, 1970).

7.   Mulligan, T., and P. G. Katz. op cit.

8.   Goldstein, I. "Overview of Types and Results of Vascular Surgical Procedures for Impotence." *Cardio Vascular and Interventional Radiology.* 11:4 (Aug 1988), 242.

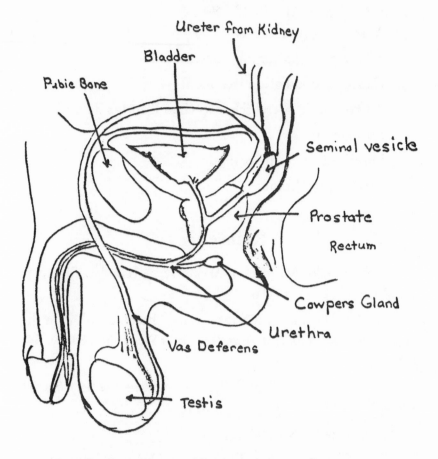

"The Urogenital System"

The Urogenital System

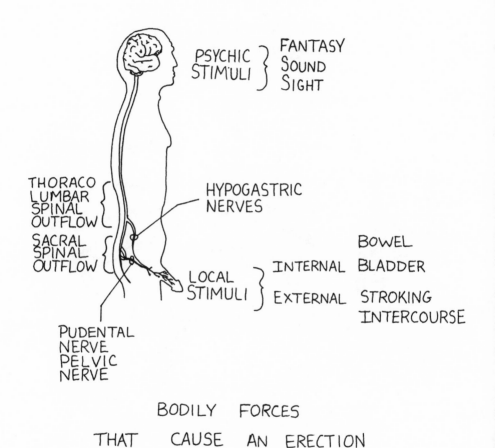

BODILY FORCES
THAT CAUSE AN ERECTION

Bodily Forces
That Cause An Erection

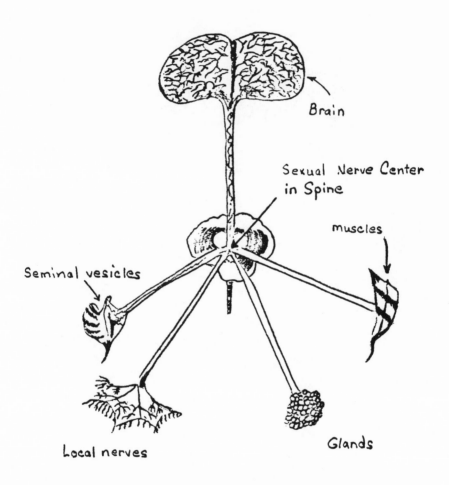

Brain

Sexual Nerve Center
in Spine

muscles

Seminal vesicles

Local nerves

Glands

" Male Sex Nerve Workings "

Male Sex Nerve Workings

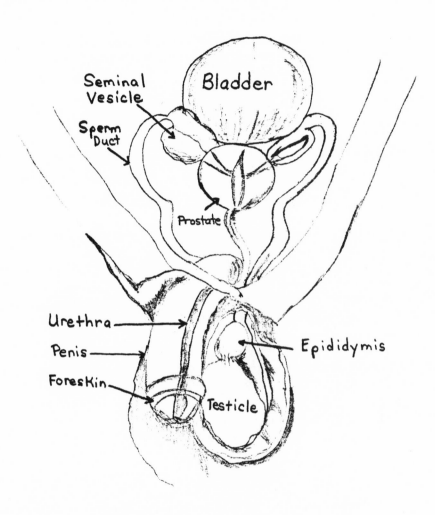

MALE   REPRODUCTIVE   SYSTEM

Male Reproductive System

Chapter 2

The Potency Killers

Arteriosclerosis

One of the major causes of insufficient blood flow to the corpora cavernosa of the penis is arteriosclerosis. Most circulatory disease is caused by narrowing of the arteries and their branches that bring blood and its life-sustaining elements throughout the body. Wherever there is blockage or impedance of blood supply to an organ, loss of function follows.

Plaques (hardened substances containing high levels of blood fats such as cholesterol) accumulate along the interior walls of the arteries, clogging them and narrowing the opening through which the blood must pass. The presence of this plaque buildup is called arteriosclerosis.

Arteriosclerosis starts with small injuries to the muscle cells that line the inner walls of the arteries. Cholesterol is considered to be the major culprit in the development of arteriosclerosis because it is a major component of plaque. Smoking and high blood cholesterol somehow erode the surfaces of blood vessels to allow more and more plaque to lay down.

If you did not clean them out these obstructions could ultimately close your arteries completely and cause heart attack, strokes, subsequent gangrene and amputation of limbs, as well as impotence. To some men's thinking, impotence is worse than heart failure!

No one who has been raised on the typical high-fat, low-fiber American diet is safe from arteriosclerosis. Over 50% of all Americans die of coronary artery disease leading to heart failure. I'm sure you have heard stories of young soldiers killed in both Korea and Viet Nam whose arteries were found to be loaded with plaque. The really shocking thing is that one study cites evidence of early signs of arterial disease in children as young as three!

Normally this killer disease develops over a period of years, but in some cases it has progressed rapidly and closed off arteries in a matter of months. Please try to understand that arteriosclerosis is not present in just one area of the body. It is a systemic condition, not a local one. For example, there are two sets of arteries supplying the brain with blood: the carotid and vertebral arteries. If either of these arteries becomes occluded and withholds blood to the brain for as little as four minutes, that person may suffer irreversible brain damage and paralysis of part of the body. Likewise, impotence can also be a symptom of arteriosclerosis. So if your penile arteries are clogged with plaque, you can be sure that this condition is found throughout your body.

Because you have arteries throughout your body, the symptoms of arterial disease manifest themselves all over your body as well. The narrowing of the arterial channels and subsequent impaired circulation can produce many of the following symptoms:

- chest pain (pectoral angina)
- vertigo and loss of balance
- partial hearing loss
- ringing in the ears

- leg pain, cramps, and tiredness

- impotence

A twenty-year medical study in Massachusetts called the Framingham Study identified three major risk factors associated with heart disease: high blood cholesterol, high blood pressure, and smoking. My method of cleansing the arteries so that they can deliver more blood to the penile arteries also corrects these pre-heart-attack conditions the natural way.

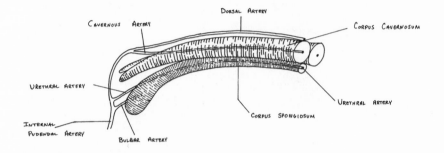

THE PENILE ARTERY AND ITS FOUR
BRANCHES

The Penile Artery and its Four Branches

Cross Section of a Clogged Artery

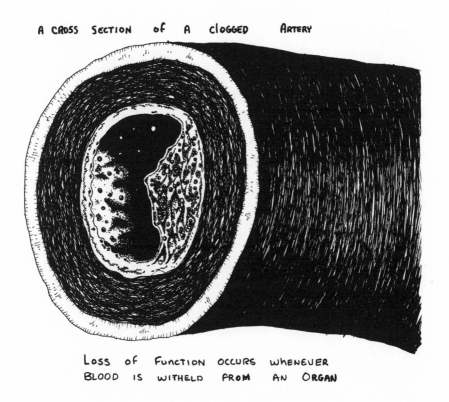

A CROSS SECTION OF A CLOGGED ARTERY

Loss of Function occurs whenever
Blood is witheld from an Organ

Loss of Function Occurs
Whenever Blood is Witheld from
an Organ

Prostate Disease:
Its Cause, Prevention and Treatment

More men suffer from prostate disease than from heart disease and cancer combined!

At least 80% of all men can expect to experience some degree of prostate trouble during their lives. Prostate disease is by no means a "disease of older men" exclusively. Yearly medical examinations are recommended after age 40.

The prostate gland is approximately the size of a walnut and surrounds the neck of the bladder and the urethra in the male. It is part gland and part muscle. The prostate secretes an opalescent, slightly alkaline fluid which forms part of the semen. Sperm makes up only a fraction of the seminal fluid and must be nourished by secretions from various glands of which the prostate is largest. These secretions activate the sperm as well as furnish them with additional nutrition for their long journey through the female reproductive tract in search of a female ovum to fertilize.

There are three main categories of prostate disease: cancer, benign prostatic hypertrophy, and prostatitis. Although perhaps as much as 99% of prostate disorders are benign, 60,000 new cases of prostate cancer are diagnosed each year, making it the second leading cause of death from cancer in American men. Prostate cancer is not uncommon in men 40 to 50 years of age. Unfortunately, most patients have advanced cancer at the time of diagnosis.[1] There are a variety of treatments for prostate cancer: complete removal of the prostate, hormone therapy with DES or other medications, radiation therapy, or radioactive implants.

Benign prostatic hypertrophy or enlargement occurs in most men who live beyond the age of 50. The symptoms include increased frequency of urination, difficulty starting the flow, dribbling and retention of urine at times. The patient may finally be unable to initiate urination at all and emergency treatment is necessary. The immediate treatment is to relieve urine buildup by a physician inserting a catheter into the bladder to drain it off. Surgery, a transurethral resection (TUR), is frequently done. Recovery is usually complete within two weeks. There are new procedures being experimented with that can relieve the symptoms without surgery such as balloon prostate dilation, which entails inserting a miniature balloon up the urethral canal and inflating it to expand the canal where it is constricted by the enlarged prostate.

Prostatitis, or inflammation of the prostate, is one of the most common prostate problems, and it may be acute or chronic. Some of the symptoms are pain during urination, blood or pus in the urine, alternating fever and chills, lower back pain, and aching joints and muscles. In chronic inflammation of the prostate, there is often diminished sex drive, partial or complete impotence, or premature ejaculation.

Causes

Although some causes of prostate disease are known, only recently has nutrition been viewed as an environmental contributor to cancer of the prostate. Recent scientific studies implicate intake of foods high in dietary fat as a major risk factor for cancer of the prostate and colon. In several major studies, incidence of prostate cancer in the United States was found to be closely related to fat consumption in the form of meat and dairy products. Other researchers have found that in the United States incidence of prostate cancer is in direct proportion to the consumption of dietary fats.[2,3,4,5]

In Japan, cancer of the prostate was almost unknown prior to 1945. However, it is now a significant disease, and the rates are still increasing because of progressive westernization of the Japanese diet.[7]

In studies of changes in prostate disease incidence in migrant workers, Haenszel and colleagues have noted that consumption of lettuce and other green vegetables and fruit appears to lower risk. There have been a number of studies which show that populations consuming a vegetarian, high-fiber diet have a much lower incidence of prostate cancer than populations consuming a Westernized diet.[8]

Diethylstilbestrol (DES) is a synthetic preparation possessing estrogenic properties, but is several times more potent than natural estrogen. It is also a known carcinogen (substance that causes cancer). In the past, it was prescribed for pregnant women to prevent miscarriages. Its usage was later linked to subsequent vaginal malignancies in daughters of women who were so treated, resulting in "DES babies." DES has also been linked to breast cancer in both females and males, benign prostatic hypertrophy, and prostate cancer. Paradoxically, it has also been used to treat prostate cancer as a kind of "chemical castration" to prolong life. However, other medications are now available that do not have all the undesirable side effects of DES.

At one time, at least 90% of all meat sold in North America came from animals that had been fed or treated with DES.[9] The purpose was to fatten the animals quickly, thus saving feed and making them available for market sooner than normal. The reaction of the animals' bodies to DES was to swell up by retaining water to dilute this toxin. This added weight to the carcasses, which was of course more profitable to ranchers.

After many years, this practice was finally outlawed because of pressure from consumer groups. How much, if any, is still being used is unknown since every animal cannot be inspected and checked for DES residues. The steroids Zeranol and Trembalone have now been legally substituted for DES in the feed of most animals raised for meat in North America.[10] Effects of all these drugs on our bodies, and particularly our prostates, may not be fully realized for years.

The point is that there is no benefit to the consumer in all of this doctoring of animal feed. The only ones who benefit are the ranchers and pharmaceutical companies.

There have been several epidemiologic studies indicating an increased risk for prostate cancer in direct proportion to an increasing number of sexual partners, prior history of venereal disease, frequency of sexual intercourse, use of prostitutes, extramarital sexual relationships, and an early age of onset of sexual activity. Together, these studies link sexual hyperactivity with excessive expenditure of seminal fluid, and promiscuity with an increased risk for prostate cancer. Additional studies demonstrate that prostatic cancer patients had more premarital and extramarital partners.[11,12,13,14,15]

Another known cause of prostate disease is lack of proper exercise, especially of the pelvic musculature. For example, it is a well known fact that pet dogs living in apartment houses who don't get sufficient exercise have a high incidence of prostate troubles, while prostate disease is almost unknown in working dogs (such as farm dogs, Eskimo dogs, and sheepdogs).

When the normal prostate enlarges because of tissue growth or swelling from inflammation, it blocks the tube leading from the bladder and cuts off free flow of urine. Symptoms that accompany prostate enlargement and congestion are widespread and varied. So, often, the underlying prostatic condition is overlooked and may be more common than is generally realized.

Since the place where pain is most severe is not necessarily the part that is the problem, it should be understood that there are limitless possibilities for wrong diagnoses. Pains emanating from the prostate are "referred pains" which manifest themselves as aches across the small of the back, pain in the hips or down the thighs, and occasionally in the abdomen.

Many patients are treated for sciatica, lumbago, sacroiliac strain, fibrositis, myositis, "honeymoon back," orchitis (inflammation of the testicles), slipped disc, phlebitis (inflammation of a vein, often associated with blood clots), cystitis, gastritis, colitis and such, when the "seat" of the pain is in the prostate.

Too often, the solution offered for prostate enlargement is to "cut it out." But about 14% of men who were potent preoperatively lose their sexual ability following a transurethral resection, and approximately 20% to 25% lose their potency after a partial prostatectomy irrespective of the surgical route: perineal, suprapubic, or retropubic.[16] Total prostatectomy almost always causes permanent impotence because the nerves and muscles to the urethra are severed.

Our Creator did not make an error when creating this organ, and "cutting it out" does not always solve the problem. Another so-called "remedy"—"medical massage" of the prostate—can be painful and irritating to the prostate and can aggravate the very condition it is supposed to correct! How this can be called a remedy, I fail to understand.

If problems with urination and referred pain are due to inflammation and swelling of the prostate, hot sitz baths taken several times daily or a hot water bottle applied to the pelvic area may help soothe inflammation and improve circulation of blood.

Your doctor may also want to give diathermy treatment (deep heat) by means of a rectal insert.

Your bowels should be kept regular by means of an enema if necessary, to relieve any pressure that may be exerted on your prostate by a ballooned colon.

The diet should be abstemious and should consist predominantly of fresh fruits of the season, green salads, and steamed vegetables. Alcohol, coffee, and spicy foods can worsen the condition.

Complete bed rest may be necessary in severe cases.

When initiation of urination becomes a problem, getting on all fours like an animal and lifting the right rear leg often helps. This is best done in the bath tub to minimize the work of cleaning up afterward.

One of the best exercises for the prostate is invisible, and takes only seconds so you can secretly perform it while you're doing dozens of daily activities. It consists of squeezing the buttocks tightly for approximately twenty to thirty seconds and then relaxing them. This exercise should be done twice a day, fifty times in the morning and fifty times in the evening. It is not even necessary to waste time while performing this exercise since many daily activities routinely performed may be done at the same time that you are performing this exercise. For instance, you can exercise while waiting for the bus or subway, waiting in line, listening to a boring person or lecture, watching TV, riding in the elevator, or even reading this book!

One of my patients, a multimillionaire from Texas, had recurrent bouts with chronic prostatitis. His prostate was swollen and tender, and he had to get up to dribble urine several times during the night. He had the usual course of "prostate massage" treatments, but it didn't help.

When he finally came to see me, I put him on a vegetarian diet, took him off coffee and alcohol, and had him temporarily discontinue sexual activity. I then prescribed a series of six exercises to be performed twice daily.

Within six weeks he was like a new man. His urinary arc was normal, he was able to sleep through the night without having to void, and he was able to resume normal sexual relations. The most effective exercise, he reported back to me, was walking on all fours like an infant, which he performed every morning for fifteen to thirty minutes. At age 80, he still does the same exercise every day, and now his employees join him!

Walking is an excellent general exercise. It aids digestion, eliminates gas, improves circulation to the prostate, and helps prevent thrombosis (blood clots) of the limbs. Slow jogging may also be beneficial for those able to do so. Isometric contractions of pelvic muscles will also help prevent these conditions.

The veins of the legs and pelvis require regular stimulation through exercise. These veins are principal sources of thrombi from which emboli may break off and lodge in distant parts of the body, incapacitating part of the lungs, causing heart failure or stroke. In 399 consecutive autopsies performed at a New York hospital, there was a 5% mortality rate due to pulmonary embolism secondary to thrombi in the legs and pelvis.[17] Another study found that thrombosis was three times as common in those who did not exercise as in those who did.

Walking is one of the best exercises you can do, but when it is not practical, try applying pressure against the footboard of the bed by alternately flexing and extending the knees.[18]

Another excellent exercise to restore circulation to the prostate is to stand with the feet apart, head back and arms spread wide. Then bend your knees, keeping your arms straight. Place your left hand on the floor and then turn your head to look at the fingertips of your right hand. Now return to the starting position and repeat with your other hand. You can find this sequence illustrated in the following section of prostate exercises.

Remember—exercise and a proper diet are not just for men who *now* suffer from prostate problems. It can help prevent the prostate problems that so many men suffer from and can help you maintain your full sexual powers for years to come.

Important Notice:

Check with your doctor before beginning any exercise, especially if you have back problems.

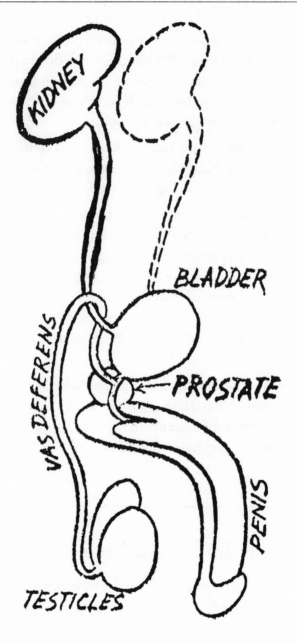

The Prostate and Bladder

Exercise for Stimulating Veins of Leg and Pelvis

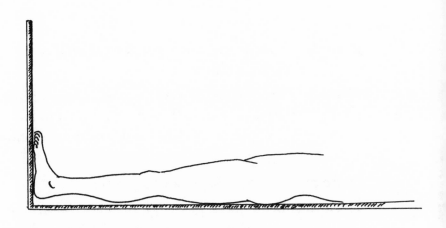

EXERCISE FOR STIMULATING VEINS OF LEG AND PELVIS

APPLY PRESSURE ON FOOTBOARD OF BED BY ALTERNATLY FLEXING AND EXTENDING KNEES

Apply Pressure on Footboard of Bed By
Alternately Flexing and Extending Knees

Exercise for Stimulating Veins

Prostate

Phase 1: Standing with feet apart, head back, arms spread wide.

Phase 2: Bending knees, keeping arms straight, place left hand flat on floor, turning head to look at fingertips of right hand, as shown in photograph.

Phase 3: Come back to starting position.

Phase 4: Bend knees, place right hand on floor, and turn to look at fingertips of left hand. Repeat. This exercise, besides benefiting the prostate, is especially prescribed for constipation or colitis.

Prostate

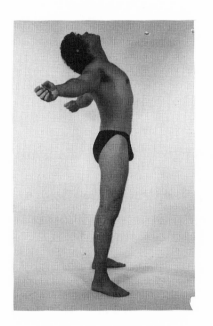 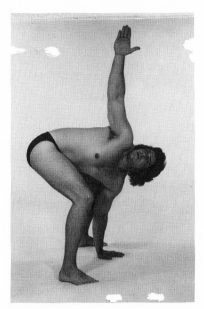

Prostate Exercises

"Spinal Stretch"
(position to encourage urination in prostatitis)

Kneeling on all fours, stretch right leg back and up as high as possible. In using this position to encourage urination in acute prostatitis, move right leg back and forth (like a dog). Do not strain. Relax. Turn on the tap water for a few minutes. Be patient. This exercise is best performed in the bathtub.

Prostate – Spinal Stretch

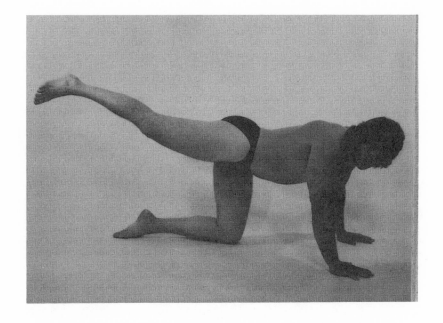

Spinal Stretch

Animal Walk Exercise

Walking on all fours like an animal. This exercise is also excellent for dropped organs (ptosis) such as your stomach. (Note: animals never have dropped organs. Neither should you.) Also for constipation, gas and other disorders of the lower intestinal tract.

Prostate

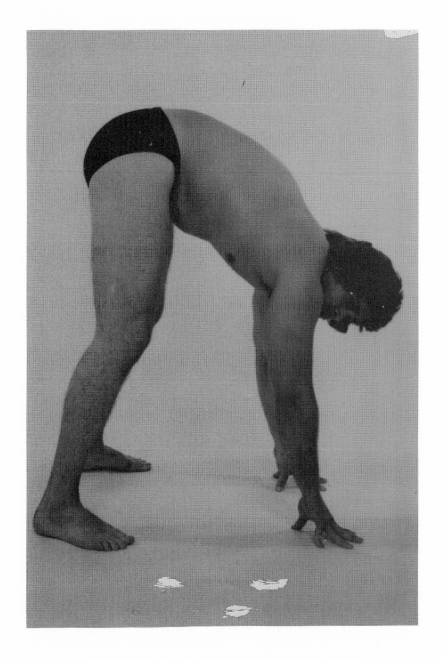

Prostate – Animal Walk Exercise

Sitting Exercise

Sitting on the floor, resting on hands, bounce right hand on cheek. Then bounce on left cheek. This exercise gives a gentle massage to the prostate and stimulates and improves blood circulation to this area.

Prostate

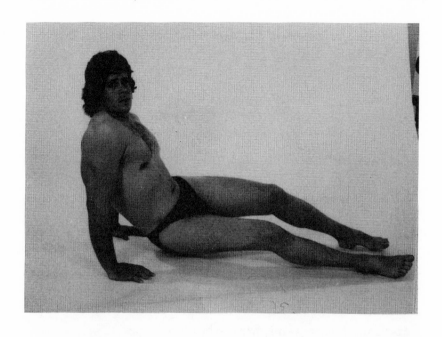

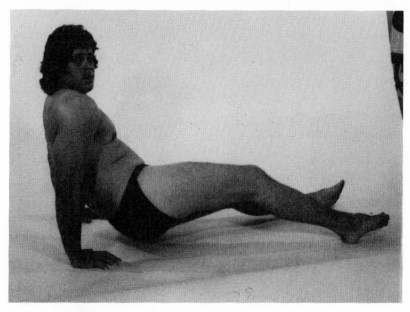

Prostate – Sitting Exercise

Abdominal Exercise

Lying on stomach, hands (fists) at sides, press fists against floor, raising legs for 10 seconds, then lower to floor. This exercise strengthens the lower back and seat muscles as well as abdominal muscles. Also for constipation, colitis, lower back weakness, varicose veins, hemorrhoids and gas.

Prostate

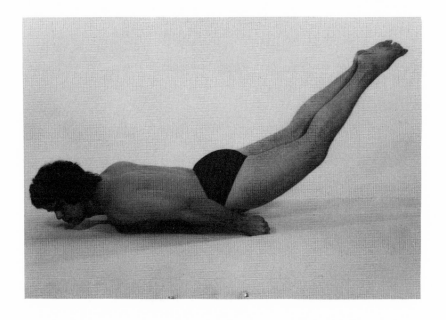

Prostate – Abdominal Exercise

High Kick

Standing with feet together, kick as high as possible, trying to touch left fingertips. Now do other side. To get the maximum benefit from these movements, you should do them without restrictive garments, or better, nude. Use also for intestinal disorders, hemorrhoids, piles, varicose veins, swollen ankles and constipation.

Prostate

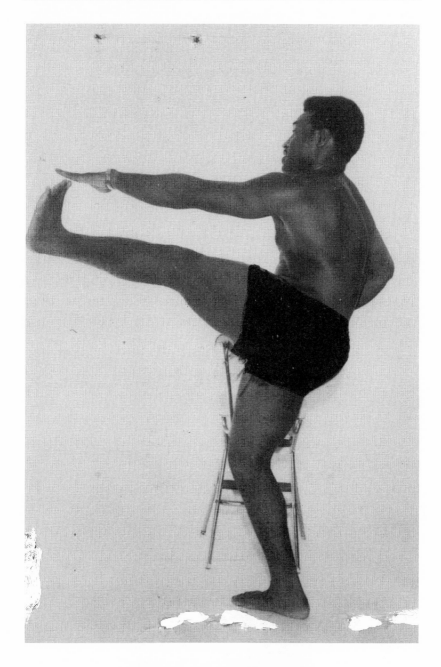

Prostate – High Kick

Bending Exercises

Standing with feet apart, knees straight, bend to touch the floor between feet. Immediately after, continuing bending body down and aim to touch floor behind you as far back as possible. Repeat as often as comfortable. Use also for waistline reducing, constipation and disorders of the lower intestinal tract.

Prostate

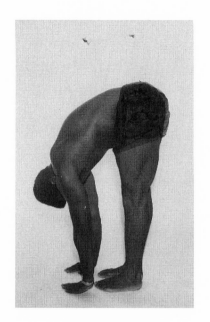 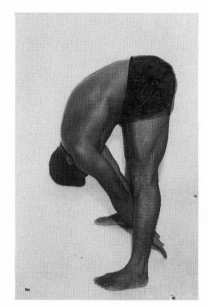

Prostate – Bending Exerciese

Bent Knee Exercise

Position 1: Standing with knees spread apart, partially bent, hands on hips as shown.

Position 2: Now lunge as far as possible to the left, inhaling deeply (as if in a fencing match). Resume position number 1, exhaling. Now do the alternate side and repeat 10 times.

Also for impotence, constipation, intestinal disorders and varicose veins.

Prostate

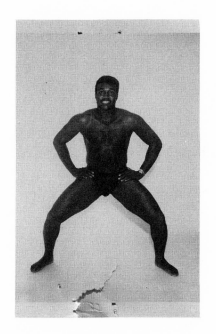
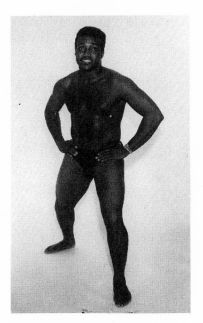

Prostate – Bent Knee Exercise

Deep Knee Bend Exercise

Position 1: Standing erect, arms overhead, holding broom handle.

Position 2: Do deep knee bend, raising heels and lowering broom handle across shoulders. Repeat. Also for intestinal stasis (constipation), intestinal disorders, prostate, congestion and varicose veins.

Impotency

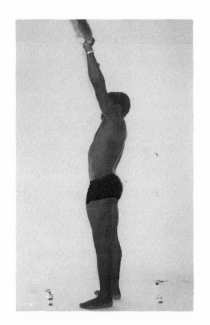 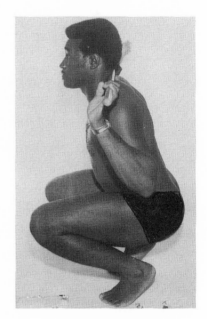

Impotency – Deep Knee Bend
Exercise

Two Impotency Exercises

Kneeling on hands and knees with arms stiff and head up, now bring head down and left knee up. Try to touch nose to knee. Return to kneeling position and repeat on alternate side.

Standing erect, feet spread widely apart, exhale and bend from trunk, touching hand to toe. Now inhale, returning to erect position. Continue same movement on opposite side. Remember to exhale while bending and inhale coming up. Repeat 10 to 20 times. Also for constipation, intestinal disorders, waistline reducing, gas, prostate trouble, and diabetes.

Impotency

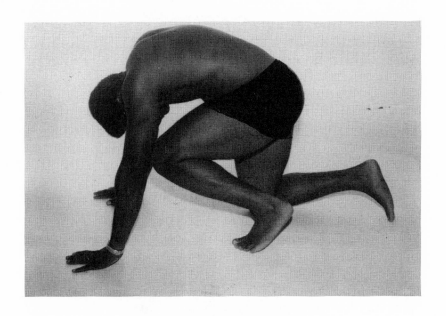

Nose to Knee Exercise

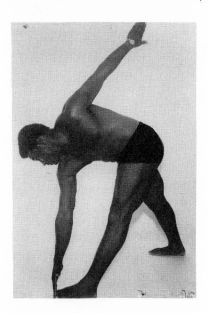

Hand to Toe Exercise

References

1. Lee, F., et al. "Prostate Cancer: Comparison of Transrectal Ultrasound and Digital Rectal Examination for Screening." *Genitourinary Radiology.* (August 1988), 389.

2. Haenszel, W., et al. "Stomach Cancer Among Japanese in Hawaii." *Journal of the National Cancer Institute.* 49 (1972), 969.

3. Schuman, L. "Epidemiology of Prostate Cancer in Blacks." *Preventive Medicine.* 9 (1980), 630.

4. Hill, P. "Environmental Factors and Breast and Prostate Cancer." *Cancer Research.* 41 (1981), 3817.

5. Blair, A., and J. F. Fraumeni. "Geographic Patterns of Prostate Cancer in the United States." *Journal of the National Cancer Institute.* 61 (1978), 1379-1384.

6. Weisburger, J. "Nutrition and Cancer—On the Mechanisms Bearing on Causes of Cancer of the Colon, Breast, Prostate, and Stomach." *Bulletin of the New York Academy of Medicine.* 56 (1980), 673.

7. Haenszel, W. *op. cit.*

8. Wynder, E. "The Dietary Environment and Cancer." *Journal of the American Dietary Association.* 71 (1977), 385.

9. Tobe, J. H. "Your Prostate". St. Catherines, Ontario, Canada: *Modern Publications,* (1967), 103-109.

10. U. S. Department of Agriculture.

11. Schuman, L., *op. cit.*

12. Steel, R., et al. "Sexual Factors in the Epidemiology of Cancer of the Prostate." *Journal of Chronic Diseases.* 24 (1972), 29-35.

13. Steel, R. "Sexual Factors in Prostate Cancer." *Medical Aspects of Human Sexuality.* 6 (1972), 70-81.

14. Krain, L. S. "Epidemiologic Variables in Prostatic Cancer." *Geriatrics.* 28 (1973), 93-98.

15. Krain, L. S. "Epidemiologic Variables in Prostatic Cancer in California." *Preventive Medicine.* 3 (1974), 154-159.

16. Thomas, W. J. "The Potency of the Ejaculatory Ducts After Prostatectomy." *British Journal of Urology.* 39 (1960), 584.

17. Morton, J. J., E. B. Mahoney, and G. B. Mider. "An Evaluation of Pulmonary Embolism Following Intravascular Venous Thrombosis." *Annals of Surgery.* 125 (1947), 590.

18. Finkle, A. L., and T. G. Moyers. "Sexual Potency in Aging Males (v) Coital Ability Following Open Perineal Prostatic Biopsy." *Journal of Urology.* 84 (1960), 152.

Medications That Can Make You Impotent

Voltaire once wrote: "Doctors are men who prescribe medicines of which they know little, to cure diseases of which they know less, in human beings of whom they know nothing." There are times, I am sorry to say, when I am inclined to agree with Voltaire.

Americans are among the most over-prescribed, over-medicated people on earth. Many patients think they are not getting their money's worth or being amply cared for unless the doctor hands them a prescription.

Drugs don't have an intelligence of their own. And drugs don't always cause the body to react the way they are supposed to and then miraculously disappear from the body. Almost every drug listed in the pharmacopoeia and the Physician's Desk Reference has side effects, adverse reactions, warnings, and contraindications. Some drugs have side effects that haven't even been discovered yet.

Patients often are too prone to depend on drugs alone to help them, rather than trying first to change their living habits. For instance, in the case of hypertension, the patient can:

1. stop smoking;

2. cut down on coffee and salt;

3. lose weight;

4. eat fewer high-cholesterol, low-fiber foods;

5. exercise more often.

Such self-applied remedies are often given second priority or ignored completely in favor of taking a hypertensive drug.

Here is a list of medications that have been reported in medical literature as causing impotence. If you are experiencing some degree of sexual dysfunction and are taking any of the drugs listed here or any other medication, do not stop taking the medication. You should report this fact to your family doctor. He or she can best evaluate your case and perhaps substitute another drug that doesn't have these side effects.

Even some over-the-counter medications, such as nasal sprays, antihistamines, and decongestants, have been reported as causing temporary impotence. It may be of interest to note that 25% of sexual problems in men were either caused by, or complicated by, medications, according to a 1983 study reported in the Journal of the American Medical Association.[1]

Drugs That Can Cause Impotence

Drugs	Possible Side Effects
Antialcoholic	
Disulfiram (Antabuse)	Erectile difficulty
Antiarrhythmic Drugs	
Disopyramide phosphate (Norpace)	Erectile difficulty
Anticholesterol	
Clofibrate (Atromid-S)	

Anticholinergics

Atropine   Erectile difficulty
Benztropine
Propantheline
Scopolamine
Trihexylphenidyl

Anticonvulsants

Carbamazepine (Tegretol)   Erectile difficulty

Antidepressant Drugs

Amitriptyline (Elavil)   Erectile difficulty, loss of
                                              libido, and ejaculatory
                                              difficulty

Desipramine (Norpramin, Pertofrane)
Doxepin (Adapin, Sinequan)
Imipramine (Janimine, Imavate, Tofranil)
Nortripyline (Aventyl, Pamelor)
Protripyline (Vivactil)
Isocarboxazid (Marplan)
Phenelzine (Nardil)
Tranylcypromine (Parnate)

Note: Nardil can also cause priapism and is the
only antidepressant to do so.

Antifungal Agents

Ketoconazole (Nizoral)   Erectile difficulty

Antihistamines

Diphenhydramine   Erectile difficulty
Hydroxyzine

Antihypertensive Drugs

Acetazolamide (Diamox)   Erectile difficulty, loss of
                                 libido, and ejaculatory
                                 difficulty
Beta Blockers (Blocaderen, Pindolol [Visken],
    Corgard, Corzide, Inderal, Lopressor,
    Acebutolol HCl [Sectral])
Clonidine (Combipres, Catapres)
Diuretics (Lozol, Zaroxolyn, Bumex, Lasix,
    Hydromox, Aldactazide, Aldactone, Edecrin)
Guanethidine (Ismelin, Esimil)
Hydralazine (Alazine, Apresoline)
Methyldopa (Aldomet, Aldoclor, Aldoril)
Pargyline (Eutonyl, Eutron)
Phenoxybenzamine
Prazosin
Propanolol
Reserpine (Serpalan, Serpasil, Diupres, Exna-R,
    Rau-Sed, Regroton, Sandril, Salutensin,
    Ser-Ap-Es)
Spironolactone
Verapamil (Calan, Isoptin)

Antipsychotic Drugs

Chlorpromazine (Thorazine)   Erectile difficulty,
ejaculatory difficulty

Fluphenazine (Prolixin)
Haloperidol (Haldol)
Lithium (Eskalith, Lithane, Lithobid, Lithonate)
Mesoridazine (Serentil)
Perphenazine (Trilafon)
Prochlorperazine (Compazine)
Thioridazine (Mellaril)
Trifluoperazine (Stelazine)

Appetite Suppressants

Amphetamine (Biphetamine)   Erectile difficulty
Chlorphentermine hydrochloride (Pre-Sate)
Fenfluramine hydrochloride (Pondimin)
Phenmetrazine (Preludin, Endurets)

Gastrointestinal Medications

Belladonna (Donnagal, Donnatal)
Cimetidine (Tagamet)   Erectile difficulty
Dicyclomine hydrochloride phenobarbital (Bentyl)
Methscopolamine (Pamine)
Metoclopramide (Reglan)
Propantheline bromide (Pro-banthine)
Tridihexethyl (Pathibamate)

Hormone Therapy for Prostate Cancer

Chlorotrianisene (Tace)
Diethylstilbestrol (Stilbestrol)

Narcotics

Cocaine   Erectile difficulty, loss of
                                         libido, and ejaculatory
                                                      difficulty

Heroin
Marijuana
Methadone
Morphine sulphate

Sedatives

Barbiturates   Erectile difficulty, loss of
                                                          libido

Chlordiazepoxide (Librium, SK-Lygen)
Diazepam (Valium)

References

1. JAMA *(Journal of the American Medical Association)*, (1983).

2. Aldridge, S. A. "Drug-induced Sexual Dysfunction." *Clinical Pharmacy* 1 (Mar-Apr 1982), 141-147.

3. Graedon, J., and T. Ferguson. "Drugs That Cause Erection Problems." *Medical Self-Care.* (Spring 1983), 54-55.

The Deadly Effects of Alcohol

Ethyl alcohol is the world's most abused drug with devastating economic and behavioral implications on society and the family. Statistics tell the story.

- There are more than twelve million alcoholics living in the United States.

- Seventy percent of the adult population consumes alcohol. But 50% of all alcohol sold is sold to 10% of drinkers.

- Out of every ten adolescents who experiment with alcohol and drugs, two of them will be addicted within twelve months.

- After 10 p.m. on a weeknight, 20% of all drivers are impaired. On a holiday weekend after 10 p.m., 25% of all drivers are impaired.

- Conservative estimates show that alcohol is involved in 50% of all homicides, 60% of all child abuse, 70% of all spousal abuse, 50% of all car crashes, and 70% of all property crime.[1,2]

- Alcohol is by far the leading drug cause of erection problems.

The deadly effects of alcohol on sexual function must have been known even in Shakespeare's time, since the porter in Macbeth says, "Drink . . .provokes the desire but takes away from the performance." Masters and Johnson, in their monumental work on human sexual inadequacy, identified alcohol as a common factor in impotence.[3]

Ethyl alcohol, generally believed to be a stimulant, is actually a depressant of the central nervous system and can cause temporary impotence when consumed even in small amounts by a social drinker. It is because alcohol, like marijuana, cocaine, and other narcotics, suppresses inhibitions that prevent a man from believing that he is the world's best lover.

It can destroy brain cells, irreparably damage the liver and pancreas, and even damage the peripheral nervous system if consumed in large amounts over many years. If damage is intense and prolonged, it can result in irreversible sexual impotence even when sober.[4]

Alcohol is also a factor in loss of sexual control or premature ejaculation. Even a couple of beers before sex can ruin a man's erection and his ejaculatory control.

Up to 80% of men who drink heavily are believed to have serious sexual problems, including impotence, sterility, and loss of sexual desire.[5] Heavy drinking over a long period of time can irreversibly destroy testicular cells, leaving men with shrunken testicles and enlarged breasts.

Alcohol also suppresses testosterone levels even in social drinkers by suppressing the secretory activity of the Leydig cells of the testicles.[6] Alcohol has many of the same undesirable pharmacological and physiological effects as nicotine. When alcohol and nicotine are introduced into the bloodstream simultaneously, the interaction of these two toxins has caused death in susceptible individuals.

Women, too, suffer from the effects of alcohol. Alcohol, even in small doses, sharply reduces a woman's sexual responsiveness as measured by photoplethysomgraphic recordings of vaginal pulse pressure and blood volume, and causes difficulty in reaching orgasm.[7] It may damage her ovaries, causing menstrual and ovulatory dysfunction and decreased estrogen production.[8] This encourages early menopause and associated signs of premature aging.

Alcohol is a teratogen, which means it can cause a deformed fetus. As little as one drink by a pregnant woman increases risk of birth defects.

There are numerous treatment centers throughout the United States and many community support groups such as Alcoholics Anonymous. The primary concern is to obtain treatment early—before the devastating effects of alcohol are permanent.

In summary, the majority of persons who commence using alcohol show little concern or knowledge about its long-term effects. Healthy nervous and circulatory systems are vital for achieving normal sexual functioning.

Alcohol can deaden nerves, impair blood circulation, and ruin your sex life. Alcohol taken simultaneously with tranquilizers, sedatives, or barbiturates is deadly. In short, alcohol can pauperize you and your family, ruin your marriage, destroy your sex life, wreck your health, and finally kill you!

References

1. Ingram, S. S. "Statistics Point the Finger at Twelve Year Olds." *Thomasville Times.* (Mar 6, 1990).

2. Liska, K. *The Pharmacist's Guide to the Most Misused and Abused Drugs in America.* (New York: Collier Books/ Macmillan, 1988), 12-13.

3. Masters, W.H., and V. E. Johnson. *Human Sexual Inadequacy.* (Boston: Little, Brown, 1970).

4. Lemere, F., and J. W. Smith. "Alcohol-induced Sexual Impotence." *American Journal of Psychiatry.* 130 (1972), 212-213.

5. Butler, R. L., and M. I. Lewis. *Love and Sex After 60.* (New York: Harper and Row, 1988), 65-66.

6. Mello, N. K. *The Pathogenesis of Alcoholism.* (New York: Plenum, 1983), 148-149.

7. Ibid.

8. Estes, N. J., and E. M. Heinemann. *Alcoholism: Development, Consequences, and Interventions.* (St. Louis: C. V. Mosby, 1977), 67-75.

Warning: Smoking Can Ruin Your Sex Life

If the surgeon general ordered cigarette manufacturers to print on their packages: *Warning: Use of this product can make a man impotent and ruin a woman's sex life,* it would be more effective in getting people to quit smoking than warning them they can get cancer or cardiovascular disease.

Advertising agencies like to portray macho-type men in their cigarette ads, implying that smoking is associated with super virility and masculinity. It may come as a surprise to 25 million male smokers that cigarette smoking can make them impotent.

Two large studies reported in the British medical journal, *The Lancet,* in 1985 that 66% of the men complaining of impotence smoked more than twice as much as the average male smoker. In another study, penile diameter changes were measured while subjects watched erotic films and smoked. The group that smoked only two cigarettes during the movie had significantly decreased penile diameters compared to the non-smokers. So smoking has both a short-term and long-term effect on potency.

Pharmacologically, nicotine constricts arteries and veins of arms and legs as well as blood vessels that supply the corpora cavernosa of the penis (two columns of erectile tissue on either side of the male sex organ). Nicotine lowers testosterone and other hormonal levels in the blood. It increases concentrations of free fatty acids in the blood, a condition that helps bring about arteriosclerosis of arteries. This further restricts blood flow to the penis and may cause impotency, especially in long-term smokers.

Tobacco can also ruin a woman's sexual function. There is evidence that smoking can interfere with ability to reach orgasm. Nicotine can damage the ovaries, causing menstrual and ovulatory abnormalities and a reduction of estrogen production, thus leading to early menopause and decreased lubrication of the vagina. Women who are on the pill have a far greater risk of dying of cardiovascular disease than nonsmokers. For example, in the 30-to-39-year age bracket of women taking the pill, the risk of developing a fatal heart attack is ten times greater in smokers. The risk of developing blood clots in the legs is also increased. Nicotine excites the nervous system at all levels and can produce tremors in the extremities. In pregnant women, smoking can damage the fetus, resulting in impaired growth and low birth weight.

The numbers of smokers have been diminishing over the years because of greater understanding of the damaging effects of nicotine on heart and lungs. Now there is another critical reason to throw away your cigarettes forever.

Reference

1.   Gilbert, D. G., R. L. Hagen, and J. A. D'Agostino. "The Effects of Cigarette Smoking on Human Sexual Potency." *Addictive Behavior.* 11 (1986), 431-434.

Psychological Causes of Impotence

In recent years, medical evidence has shown us that only about 40% to 50% of impotence is due to psychological causes. Loss of sexual potency is not a natural consequence of aging, but may be an indication of physical disease or unrealistic psychological expectations in our culture.

In their book, *It's Not All in Your Head*, Bruce and Eileen MacKenzie list signs of psychogenic impotence:

- If the onset of your impotence was sudden, perhaps after the death of a spouse or following another life crisis, then you may be experiencing *temporary* impotence. Your situation may resolve itself after a short recovery period or some counseling. If not, proper evaluation may indicate chronic psychogenic impotence.

- If you can have sex with some partners and not with others, you are probably suffering from psychogenic impotence.

- If you have erections during your sleep, you may have psychogenic impotence. (This may be misleading, because your nighttime erections might last only thirty seconds or so rather than thirty to forty minutes, possibly indicating a physiological problem.)

- If you can masturbate and maintain an erection through ejaculation, again, you are probably psychogenically impotent.

The psychological factors affecting potency include per-formance anxiety, depression, stress and anxiety, relationship deterioration, guilt feelings over an extramarital affair, bore-dom, and loss of interest (often interpreted as impotence).

The most common causes of psychogenic impotence are performance anxiety and depression. If a man is tired or worried about something, he may have a temporary problem getting an erection. The next time he tries to make love, his concern that he will have problems again can cause another failure. Some-times this goes away quickly if the partner is understanding; however, if the problem persists beyond several weeks, a visit to a doctor or psychological counselor may be necessary. Once he realizes that his impotence is only temporary, the problem usually goes away.

Depression is also a common cause of sexual dysfunction. It may come on gradually or suddenly because of a dissatisfac-tion with life. Depression frequently causes a loss of interest in sex. Treatment may be psychological counseling or medication. Unfortunately, many medications used to treat depression also cause impotence as side effects. It is important that the depres-sion be evaluated by a psychiatrist before it becomes long-standing.

Men may have psychogenic impotence after going through an illness, such as a heart attack. Most doctors allow their patients to resume sex four to six weeks after a heart attack if there are no contraindications.

Many people gain weight and are less attractive to their partners, perhaps ashamed of themselves and reluctant to be nude, even with their spouses. This can cause a loss of libido and temporary impotence in either or both partners.

Marital discord, or relationship deterioration, can cause both impotence and lack of interest in sex. When two people are arguing all the time, they have little interest in sharing the intimacy of lovemaking. Once potency fails, many women react with resentment or disappointment. Others may buy new clothes or lingerie to try to become more sexy, thinking that they are the cause of the problem. Often these efforts to be more alluring just put more pressure on the man. The woman may feel she is unloved or suspect that he is having an affair. These destructive behaviors must be dealt with if the relationship is to continue. Treatment may involve marital counseling and sex therapy.

Sex Therapy

Sex therapy programs involve psychological counseling and instruction in methods to improve communication skills and sexual techniques. Some sex therapy programs work only with couples; others accept single people for treatment. Programs may be concentrated into two weeks or may be extended up to three months with visits for treatment once a week. Contrary to popular belief, a sex therapist never has sex with the clients or observes them making love.

There is a strong emphasis on improving communication in the relationship. Research shows that in order to have a successful relationship, these factors are important:

- Affection—a sense of genuine concern for the other person.

- Expressivity—the ability to share and be vulnerable, a willingness to be open and honest about feelings and needs, not just those that are sexual but covering all human concerns.

- Sexuality—this is a positive interest in sex, the opposite of inhibited desire.

- Commitment—an honest sense of trust in the other person and a notion of permanency about the relationship.

- Compatibility—having shared interests, at least to a reasonable degree.

- Conflict resolution—the ability to resolve differences and conflicts as they arise without creating overwhelming tension.

- Autonomy—an ability to live alone as well as with one's spouse. This is the opposite of complete dependence.

Masters and Johnson developed a form of treatment called sensate focus therapy for treating psychological impotence. They claim a 74% success rate in curing impotence of less than one year standing in couples where there is no depression or hostility. However, sensate focus therapy is not effective in treating loss of libido. Some examples of sensate focus exercises are given in Chapter 8.

Surrogate partners are women and men trained in using sensate focus exercises to help people with sexual dysfunction. They are not prostitutes. Their role is to be supportive and to guide the patient in the use of these exercises to regain the pleasures of sex.

A list of sources to help you find a sex therapist is given in back of the book.

Other Treatments

Hypnosis is sometimes used to treat impotence from psychological causes to relieve unconscious fears and anxiety.

Acupuncture is used to treat impotence by inserting and rotating needles in the lower portion of the abdomen and near the ankle.

Biofeedback to relieve tension and anxiety may help resolve underlying causes of psychological impotence. A machine is attached to a part of the patient's body, usually the forehead, and the patient learns to control muscular tension by listening to the rising and falling sound the machine makes as the muscles contract and relax.[3]

References

1. MacKenzie, Bruce and Eileen. *It's Not All in Your Head.* (New York: E. P. Dutton, 1988), 14-15.

2. Skalka, P. *Guide to Health and Well-Being After Fifty.* (New York: Random House, 1984), 140.

3. Brooks, Marvin. *Lifelong Sexual Vigor.* (Garden City, NY: Doubleday, 1981), 181-182.

Constipation: The Root Of Impotency And Disease . . .
And How To Finally Cure It

Men who want to achieve their optimal level of sexual potency must learn to deal effectively with the common problem of constipation, which plays a primary role in impotence.

More people suffer from constipation than any other ailment, and the same lack of common sense shown in treatment centuries ago is still used today. Witness the hundreds of "remedies" offered in every drugstore, recommended constantly on television and radio commercials and in newspaper ads.

In spite of all the claims, most of the "cures" actually worsen the condition they are supposed to correct, and none of them removes the basic cause of the problem. The usual treatment displays chronic *intellectual* constipation of years standing.

You must realize that not only impotence is made worse by constipation, but also diseases of your kidney, urinary tract, uterus, circulation, digestion, lungs, blood, intestines, or rectum.

Millions of people consume laxatives as though they were chewing gum or eating candy. In fact, some laxatives *are* candy or chewing gum. In the United States in 1987 Americans spent over 366 million dollars on laxatives. Many of these laxatives are irritating to the delicate lining of the stomach and intestines, remove valuable fluids from the blood, afford only temporary relief at best, and tend to be habit-forming.

One of the main consequences of the laxative habit is that it teaches the practice of palliating symptoms, not removing causes. It makes a person more and more dependent upon the laxative habit in order to force the bowels to move, instead of getting at the root of the problem. In summary, it worsens the condition it is supposed to correct.

Constipation is not a disease as commonly defined, but rather an effect due to improper living habits. It is the forerunner of many diseases. It is not caused by germs or any other external entity, but occurs through a deliberate course of action or inaction which is contrary to the body's natural order.

The high-protein, high-fat, low-fiber, highly processed American diet, lack of proper exercise, improperly sitting for long periods of time on chairs that are built too high off the ground, incorrect toilet habits on toilets that are improperly designed, and stress are all factors in creating our most prevalent basic health problem—constipation. Rather than changing or eliminating the aforementioned bad habits that have caused this condition in the first place, most people prefer to grasp, like drowning men, at every straw.

They have tried enemas, mineral oil, bran, prune juice, suppositories, bulking agents, phenolphthalein, and all the other expedients advertised. And they are *still* constipated!

There is a law of cause and effect that says you cannot cure a disease without first removing its cause, or another disease must follow. If all you do is take enemas, use mineral oil, bran, prune juice, etc., and continue eating the wrong foods and not exercising properly, you are fooling only yourself. You must get at the roots of this problem.

Health cannot be bought; it must be built!

Americans spend more money on drugs and surgery than any other country in the world. Still, approximately one out of every four Americans will develop cancer and 400,000 of them will die this year. One out of every two Americans dies of coronary artery disease. Seventy-seven percent of our adult population has arthritis. Eighty percent of men will suffer from prostate disease. One out of four Americans suffers from hypertension. Ten million American children are mentally retarded.

The point is that if we are spending more money on drugs and surgery than any other country in the world, shouldn't it follow logically that if what we are doing is correct, we would also be the healthiest country in the world? But in terms of longevity, we are number twenty from the top. Even countries like Puerto Rico that spend far less on hospitals, surgery, and drugs have higher longevity rates than the United States.

Constipation is an effect due to wrong living habits. And the only honest cure for wrong living habits is to develop right ones. If a man is standing on hot coals and is in pain, do you offer him a couple of aspirin to suppress the pain or do you tell him to get off the hot coals first?

A person cannot be constipated in just one part of the body without it affecting other areas of the body. There is a unity of all things, including human disease. A man's body cannot function at peak efficiency and be responsive sexually if it is clogged and polluted with uneliminated wastes.

Some people have the mistaken idea that they can "clean themselves out" by taking a laxative like a plumber cleans out a sewer. The human colon is not like a sewer pipe; it is not made of cast iron.

That their bodies need cleaning out is true. Few people are truly clean on the inside although they may appear very clean on the outside. If we are to regard our bodies as "temples of our souls," then we would certainly not want to desecrate these temples with garbage.

Our bodies, like automobiles, were designed to operate most efficiently on a certain type of fuel. An automobile is designed to operate on gasoline; if necessary, it can be made to run on kerosene, but it will not run as efficiently. The motor will get clogged with carbon and other exhausts and stop functioning efficiently long before its life expectancy.

Your body is designed to operate most efficiently on a low-fat, mostly vegetarian diet. It can, if necessary, be made to run on the rich, high-fat, high-protein, low-fiber typical American diet. However, like the car, it will not operate as efficiently. It will get clogged up with toxic wastes and stop functioning properly long before its life expectancy.

Laxatives are not part of the solution; they are part of the problem.

Enemas are not the answer either. Our bodies were not designed to have water or any other substance injected into the rectum. Enemas and colonics distend and stretch the colon, reduce its elasticity, remove beneficial intestinal flora, wash away part of the protective mucus lining, and may further irritate an already irritated colon. In short, in the long run, it tends to make the condition worse.

Mineral oil is also not the answer. Mineral oil coats the lining of the intestines, stopping absorption of fat-soluble vitamins and minerals.

Phenolphthalein, a common ingredient in many laxatives, is obtained by the interaction of phenol (a distillate of coal tar, and dangerous because of its corrosive action on tissues) and phthalic anhydride. The body draws large quantities of water from the blood in order to dilute this toxin, and then flushes it out through the intestines. This causes dehydration of the body. The person taking this substance believes he is "getting cleaned out," when actually the body intelligence is flushing this poison out through the rectum as fast as it can get rid of it.

Bran is another "remedy." It is well known that lack of "bulk" or indigestible fiber in the diet contributes to intestinal stasis, or constipation. Lack of sufficient fiber in the diet is also a contributing factor in the etiology of cancer of the colon. Bran is now being heavily promoted as a commercially expedient solution to the problem. In my experience, bran can be particularly disastrous. I have witnessed it turn some people into permanent invalids when habitually used.

What is bran? Bran is part of the whole wheat kernel after it has been separated from the flour. In my opinion, it was a serious mistake to separate the two in the first place. Bran is composed mainly of the indigestible fiber, or cellulose, part of the wheat, and is usually too rough on the intestines for human consumption.

Eating whole wheat is fine and normal, but to separate one particular element from a whole natural food is against the normal order of things and can be harmful in the long run. It is what we call a fractionated food.

I, as well as many of my colleagues, have often been kept busy treating colitis cases (colons so irritated they had to have five to twenty movements a day) because of eating bran over an extended period of time as a means of curing their constipation.

How then can a person become clean on the inside, super potent at any age, and maintain a pure bloodstream? By eating the foods nature intended for us to eat, exercising properly, and getting rid of bad living habits!

Of all the crimes we commit aginst nature, our eating practices are probably the worst offenders. The basic premise most people use as a criterion for their nutrition is, "If it tastes good, it's good for you." I might go along with this premise if food were eaten in its natural, unadulterated, unseasoned, and uncooked state and if our taste buds were not perverted through habit and years of conditioning.

Most of us are slaves to the "great god of taste." However, taste is largely a matter of habit or conditioning. Let me give you some examples. If you were born an Eskimo, whale blubber and polar bear dung would taste delicious! If you were born a Zulu, drinking the blood of cattle would be a normal meal. If you happened to be raised a cannibal, you wouldn't have second thoughts about having your fellow man for dinner.

The point is: from the moment we are born, we become creatures of habit; and habit, in man, can surmount reason. After habit has become second nature, we lose awareness of what we are doing, regardless of the consequences of our actions. Humans long ago lost the sense of taste as an effective protection from harmful food. Additionally, commercial food processors have added sweeteners, chemicals and preservatives and pervert our sense of taste. Therefore we can no longer rely on our taste buds to act as a guide to protect us from harmful food.

The basic principle of all nutrition is, or should be, the less tampering with natural food the better. If we follow this principle, we are on the right track. Most European countries prohibit by law the artificial coloring and flavoring of food merely for deception.

Judging from labels on most canned foods, TV dinners, and other prepared foods, the average person is eating a mouthful of chemicals from which his body tries to manufacture living tissue.

Like the superior and inferior types of fuel that the automobile can use, humans also have two categories of fuel on which to run their bodies. These two are "live food" and "dead food."

Dead food is all food that no longer possesses life force. It no longer contains oxygen, enzymes, or bioelectricity—in short, the essence of life. All cooked and canned food is dead. Living food is uncooked, for example, fresh fruits, raw vegetables and uncooked nuts. All dead food is obstructive and is in various stages of decomposition, encouraging fermentation.

For example, Robert Rodale reported that "the Abkhasians in Russia, some of whom live to be over 125 years old, routinely perform their marital functions to the age of one hundred. The Hunzas become parents at advanced ages, and so do the residents of Vilcabamba, that mountain valley in Ecuador known for the extreme old age its residents reach. There is no reason why we can't adapt our lifestyles to gain the health advantages these remarkable people enjoy."

How is it done? There are no tricks, no aphrodisiacs. Even if true aphrodisiacs did exist, how could they stimulate your sexual function past the age of 100, if illness had snuffed out your life at 55? We can only look at the way of life these long-living, sexually active people follow, and see what we can copy.

"The Abkhasians have an abhorrance of stale food. Everything is prepared fresh for each meal. Members of all three long-lived societies eat much less than we do, and their food is simple and unprocessed. Yet, despite meager diets, they work harder physically. Their bodies are lean and hard, not larded with fat."

Uncooked foods transport oxygen and oppose putrefaction. They are vitalized with living enzymes to aid digestion. Cooked starch, refined sugar, and animal proteins tend to ferment or undergo putrefaction relatively rapidly.

Cooked oils or fats are particularly harmful. Whenever any oil or fat is heated above body temperature, it becomes a carcinogen, a substance that produces or incites cancer.

Most foods sold in franchise establishments—so-called "fast food restaurants"which serve hamburgers, cheeseburgers, fried chicken and fried fish and chips that are so well-patronized provide excellent future business for cancer specialists. Most of these restaurants cook their foods using animal fat or cooking oil that has been heated to a high temperature and kept there. The oil or grease is often black, and the same oil is often used day in and day out—sometimes week in and week out. Is it surprising that 25% of the American people die of cancer?

One other word of warning—about appetite. Man's appetite is fickle and easily deceived. "Whatever tastes good is good for you" is a most unreliable guide. Man, unlike the lower animals, cannot rely on instinct, but must depend on his brains and power of reasoning to guide him to correct eating patterns.

What types of food should you avoid? If you deliberately wanted to make someone constipated, sick and impotent, what type of foods would you feed him? Foods that make paste and clog up his arteries, of course! What are these foods? Here is a partial list of the main offenders:

Flour and water make paste. This includes "enriched" bread, white bread, and doughnuts. Anything "enriched" has first to be impoverished. Whole wheat has twenty-four natural vitamins and minerals. The commercial millers remove *all* of these natural vitamins and minerals in order to lengthen "shelf life" and make the product whiter. They then put back four synthetic vitamins. What or who is being enriched?

Pastry is paste. This includes Danish pastries, French pastries, Italian pastries, etc. Every country has its own brand of paste.

Baked paste includes pizza, flan, pies, cakes, custards and cookies. Delicious?   Perhaps, but they make you fat and constipated.

Milk products make paste. Casein, one of the components of cow's milk (not present in human mother's milk) is used in the manufacture of paste. In fact, one of the largest manufacturers of paste is also one of the leading processors of milk. All pasteurized or cooked milk products are constipating. Since the farmer gets paid by the butterfat content of the milk, cows are fed and bred with the purpose of increasing the fat content of their milk. Whole milk today is about 4% fat by weight, but has almost half its calories in fat. Most of that fat is saturated, the type that increases blood cholesterol levels, clogs up your arteries, and promotes heart disease and impotence.

Eggs make paste. Eggs are used in a recipe in order to "bind" the ingredients together. Eggs, like meat, fish, and milk products, have zero fiber content. The chicken and cow are the most exploited of all animals. Eggs have one of the highest cholesterol levels of any food. The chickens get even with people who eat their eggs by clogging their arteries and killing them with arteriosclerosis and heart disease.

White rice makes excellent paste for bookbinders. It's called rice paste. It also helps bind your intestines. Almost all vitamins and minerals are also removed when they remove the bran. None of this applies to brown rice or to rice which hasn't had the bran removed.

Meat, fish, and poultry. These foods putrefy rapidly in the intestines, are high in uric acid, contribute to clogging arteries with cholesterol, and have zero fiber content. They contribute to colon cancer and constipation.

Cocoa. All cocoa and chocolate products contain the toxin theobromine, a chemical cousin of caffeine, and the body reacts similarly to both. Cocoa is constipating and is high in saturated fat.

Coffee contains the toxin caffeine, a stimulant and irritant to the stomach, intestines, and urinary tract. Coffee is therefore a factor in intensifying irritation to these and other body organs and should be eliminated when these organs are weakened by disease.

When we consider that most people consume tremendous quantities of these pasty and obstructive foods daily as the mainstay of their diets, we understand why the most common medical complaints are delayed elimination (constipation) and clogged arteries (arteriosclerosis). In fact, it is axiomatic that the degree of constipation and clogged arteries, as well as all other abnormal conditions arising because of constipation and clogged arteries, is in direct ratio to the paste and cholesterol in one's diet. Too often that seven-course meal turns into a seven *curse* aftermath!

Next to incorrect eating habits and improper sitting posture, lack of proper exercise is the leading cause of constipation and associated diseases such as colitis, varicose veins, hemorrhoids, gas and indigestion. The abdominal muscles, which are intended to support the abdominal and visceral organs as well as the intestinal corset, are weakened and lack tone because of insufficient exercise and poor sitting and standing posture. This weakness or lack of muscle tone causes a ptosis, or drooping of these organs, as well as a sagging of the transverse colon, until they almost touch the pelvic floor at times. Obesity can be a factor in causing this condition. The only method of strengthening weak muscles is through exercise. No one can have good muscle tone without exercise.

The first key to a trouble-free digestive system, unflagging energy, regular bowel movements, and a healthy functioning of the sexual apparatus is to develop strong abdominal and eliminative muscles. Every time we eat, peristaltic action begins and continues along the entire digestive tract, from the esophagus to the anus. Ideally, a person should move his bowels after every meal.

Plato once said that all diseases can be cured by proper exercise and diet. The only exception to this, of course, is when the digestive organs are so debilitated that they require rest before any other treatment. In very debilitated cases, passive exercises and massage may be best.

General exercise, within reason, stimulates all functions of the body; secretions and excretions will stay normal in most people who lead active lives.

However, as I mentioned before, eating proper food, getting the proper rest, and thinking positively and optimistically must all be taken into consideration. Some books are just for reading and for passing the time. This book is for study and practice, so you can enjoy your life more through better health.

The ensuing exercises may lack the spectacular thrills of modern medical science, but those who prefer the thrills and frills of needless operations with gradually worsening health can pay their money and take their choice.

The persons who invented modern toilets and chairs never realized the havoc they were to cause our bodies in the form of constipation, prostate disorders, hemorrhoids, varicose veins, and related diseases by designing them too high off the ground. In addition to prostate disorders and constipation, the sitting position and the chair are important factors in causing venous thrombosis embolism. The usual sitting position using a chair induces thrombosis of the popliteal veins by sharply angulating valves in the calves of the legs, therby promoting vascular clots, varicosities and intestinal stasis.

Our bodies were not designed for us to sit on chairs. They were designed for us to squat. The "Supreme Engineer" intended, when creating the human body, that it should be used properly. Most primitive peoples instinctively squat or sit on a low stool or bench while eating, resting, or defecating. And prostatic diseases and constipation are extremely rare among these people.

I have instructed many of my patients in the natural and proper way to sit on a toilet by putting a stool on which they place their feet directly in front of the toilet. This simple correction, without need of any further treatment, gave a much more complete evacuation and enabled many to overcome even severe constipation.

Here is a simple test of the benefits of squatting. Next time you sit on the toilet, after you think you have finished evacuating in your usual position, raise your legs, placing the feet on the toilet seat or a stool. Wait a few moments and then notice the additional quantity of stool passed after assuming the latter position. This should convince anyone of the benefits derived from squatting or raising the legs while defecating.

Constipation Exercises

Standing erect, feet apart, knees slightly bent, lean forward with hands on thighs as shown. Exhale completely, pulling abdominal muscles in. This exercise should only be performed on an empty stomach, preferably before breakfast.

FOR ADVANCED STUDENTS ONLY: While holding position, and without inhaling, try rotating abdominal muscles first to the right and then to the left. While this exercise is intended for advanced students, it is certainly one of the most effective movements for constipation and dropped abdominal organs.

Constipation

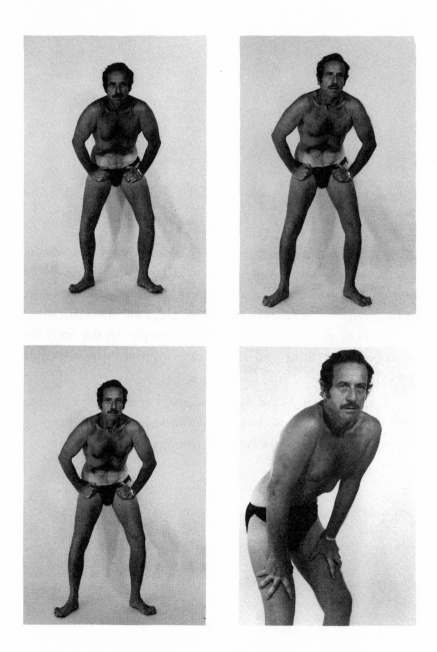

Constipation Exercises

Slant Board Exercises

Lying on slant board, with legs higher than head, resting on elbows and hips. Now raise hips as high as possible. Then lower hips slowly to board and repeat as often as comfortable. In addition to constipation and disorders of the lower intestinal tract, this exercise is also beneficial for preparing the body for natural childbirth as well as for restoring the internal organs after childbirth.

Lying on slant board, feet strapped, hands in back of neck with fingers interlaced, twist to left side from waist keeping buttocks on board. Now twist all the way to the right side.

Constipation

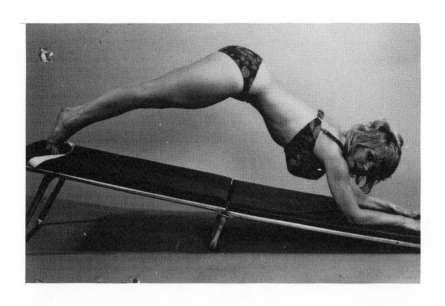

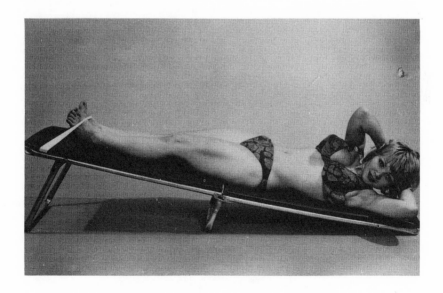

Constipation - Slant Board
Exercises

Slant Board Twist Exercises

Lying on slant board, feet strapped, raise trunk, twisting to the left, then, swinging arms as shown, twist to right. Keep alternating left to right as long as there is no undue strain.

Constipation

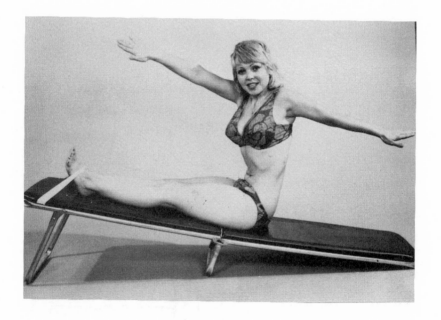

Slant Board Twist Exercise

How Sitting On A Chair Can Be
Hazardous To Your Health

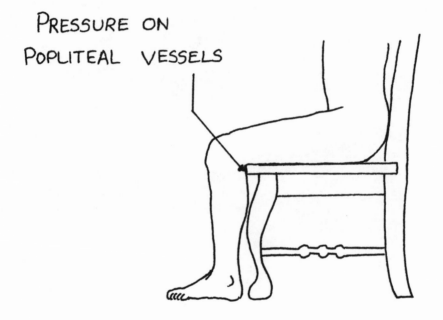

PRESSURE ON
POPLITEAL VESSELS

Sitting in a Chair

References

1. *The Nielsen OTC/HBA Index for 1987. Drug Topics.* (April 18, 1988).

2. Kurian, G. *New Book of World Rankings.* (New York: Facts on File Publications, 1986).

3. *Demographic Year Book.* (New York: National Center for Health Statistics).

4. Rodale Robert. *The Best Health Ideas I Know.* (Emmaus, PA: Rodale Press, 1974), 10.

5. *The American Medical Association Family Medical Guide.* J.R. Kunz, M.D., editor. (New York: Random House, 1982), 306-7.

6. Roman, R.L. *Sex and the Unborn Child.* (New York: Julian Press, 1969).

7. Breggin, Peter Roger, M.D. *Psychiatric Drugs: Hazards to the Brain* (New York: Springer, 1983), 180-1, 93-9, 25-8, 194.

Chapter 3

Aphrodisiacs – And Why I Think They're Unnecessary

SINCE ANCIENT TIMES MAN HAS SEARCHED FOR aphrodisiacs to enhance desire and sexual performance. A few substances used as aphrodisiacs are ground rhinocerous tusk, garlic, prunes, artichokes, oysters, and truffles. There is no evidence that any of these affect anything except the imagination.

Spanish fly has a reputation as a potent aphrodisiac because it irritates the digestive system and urinary tract, causing a painful erection that is unrelated to sexual arousal. Its side effects include vomiting, diarrhea, shock and even death.[1]

Marijuana has often been touted as intensifying the sexual act through sensory enhancement, prolongation of time sense, increased fantasy imagery, and a decrease in inhibition. However, in a study in 1980, daily marijuana users were found to have intercourse 80% less often than the control group, with 40% less frequency of orgasms. Female users had shorter and more irregular menstrual cycles. Long-term use of marijuana is known to cause loss of libido as well.[2]

Vitamin E is another alleged aphrodisiac, but there is no scientific evidence to back this claim.

Amyl nitrate and isobutyl nitrate, or poppers, are heart medications that reportedly cause intensified orgasm and heightened awareness during sex. They are taken by breaking open a capsule and inhaling the vapors. Side effects are low blood pressure, headaches, rapid pulse rate, nausea, and dizziness.[3]

111

Many herbal enthusiasts believe that ginseng enhances sex drive, contrary to the mainstream medical community, who remain skeptical. However, recent reports by two British physicians, Drs. B.V. Palmer and O.M. Koriech, may give more credence to these assertions. The doctors reported an increase in sexual responsiveness and breast enlargement in females taking ginseng and hypothesized that these effects were a result of increased hormonal activity brought about by the ginseng. There was no mention of the effects of ginseng on men.[4]

Tryptophan is an amino acid that has been used as an over-the-counter medication for its sedative effects, and as a prescription drug for schizophrenia. It has also been noted to cause increased sexual desire. The FDA has recalled all tryptophan recently. However, it is expected that it will be getting a clean bill of health and should be available soon.

Beware advertising claims selling "pills for potency." These often cause urethral irritation and allergic reactions.

Prescription Medications

Since the 1960s doctors have noted that some prescription drugs can cause heightened sexual interest. Patients taking L-dopa for Parkinson's disease have reported increased sex drive.

The drugs parachlorophenylalanine (PCPA) and apomorphine HCl have been experimentally shown to increase sexual desire. Luteinizing hormone-releasing hormone (LHRH) also intensifies sexual activity, especially when combined with estrogen in women and testosterone in men. None of these medications are currently being used to treat impotency or loss of libido.[5]

There are new medications that appear to be effective in helping impotent men achieve erections for sexual intercourse. All require prescriptions and have no effect on orgasm or ejaculation.

Yohimex or Yocon are trade names for yohimbine, an alkaloid derived from trees indigenous to Africa, and are taken orally. Yohimbine has been identified by medical researchers as an alpha-2 adrenergic blocking agent useful in diagnosis and treatment of some types of erectile dysfunction. It is also used as a mydriatic agent (to dilate the pupil of the eye) and as a sympathicolytic (to interefere with, oppose, or destroy impulses from the sympathetic nervous system). Yohimbine readily penetrates the central nervous system, producing peripheral sympathetic nerve blocking. This theoretically results in increased penile blood flow.[6,7,8]

In experimental doses of the drug to treat impotence, one tablet (5.4 mg.) was given three times a day to adult males. Occasional side effects reported at this dosage are nausea, dizziness, or nervousness.

Papaverine, either alone or combined with phentolamine, works by dilating the blood vessels of the penis to allow increased blood flow to the erectile tissues. The drug is injected directly into the penis and cannot be used more than twice a week. It is deemed effective for both psychological and physiological impotence. Papaverine, which is a smooth muscle relaxant, can induce erections rigid enough to permit intercourse in 81% to 100% of all impotence types.

Dr. Roger E. Nellans, a urologist at the University of Washington, gave injections of papaverine to 75 selected patients suffering from both psychological and physiological impotence. He reported that the average duration of the erections was three-and-a-half hours. Papaverine has been described as "a lifeline for (impotent) patients, eliminating performance anxiety and helping them regain their self-esteem."[9]

However, before you rush down to your urologist and demand a papaverine injection, there are some "risks, possible complications, and undesirable side effects." One of the risks reported is that of developing a priapism—an abnormal erection of very long duration—which can cause fibrosis of the penis and permanent impotence.

Dr. Michael A. Perlman, clinical professor of psychiatry at Cornell University, reports that a patient who developed priapism after an injection of papaverine subsequently had "diminished erectile function that was worse than before treatment." Other possible side effects are fibrosis of the penis at the injection site, orthostatic hypotension (low blood pressure upon rising), and bruising.

Dr. Nellans acknowledges that the therapy has "definite medical and legal risks." However, if everything else has failed, you may want to discuss papaverine injections or other drug therapy with your physician. Although neither the FDA nor the drug manufacturer approves it for injection into the penis, papaverine is being administered by doctors throughout the United States with proper informed consent. Once the physician and patient decide that trial treatments have been successful, the patient is trained to give his own injections at home.

Other drugs being used to induce erections after direct injection into the penis are vasoactive intestinal peptide, prostaglandin-E, and nitroglycerin. Vasoactive intestinal peptide is an amino acid group that triggers nerve transmitters to increase blood flow to the penis. Prostaglandin-E is less caustic than papaverine and has fewer side effects, but costs three times as much. Nitroglycerin can be either injected directly into the penis or applied topically with a 2% cream to increase local blood flow. Studies are being done to develop effective oral medications from these drugs.

Another kind of treatment is testosterone replacement therapy. Testosterone is given once or twice a week for six weeks. If it is effective, the patient goes on a maintenance program of one dose every four to six weeks. Potential side effects are increased risk of liver and prostate cancer, chemical hepatitis, water retention, and high blood pressure.

I want to emphasize that any man taking any of these drugs should be under the care of a physician. I hope this book enables you to achieve your maximal potency without drugs.

Keep in mind that every drug in the entire pharmacopoeia has "side effects," some known, some unknown. And drugs usually fail to deal with correcting or removing the real cause of the problem, ignoring the law of cause and effect. Therefore drugs can be dangerous, addictive, unpredictive and certainly less effective than other methods, including changing your life-style, as suggested elsewhere in this book.

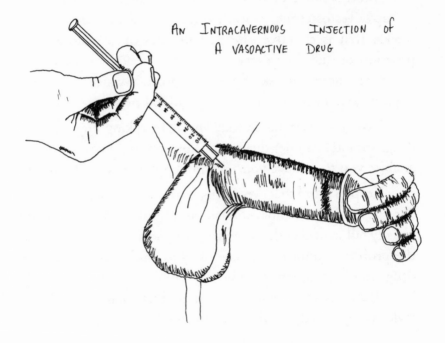

An Intracavernous Injection of a
Vasoactive Drug

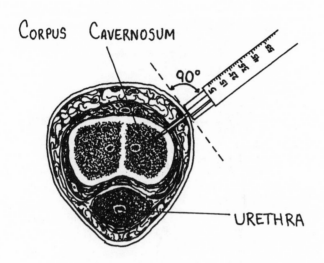

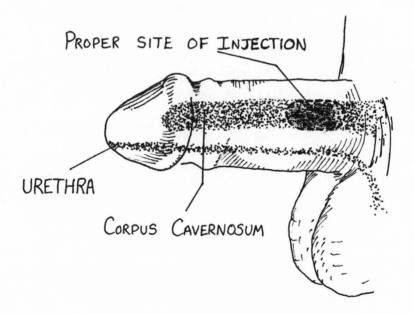

Proper Site of Injection

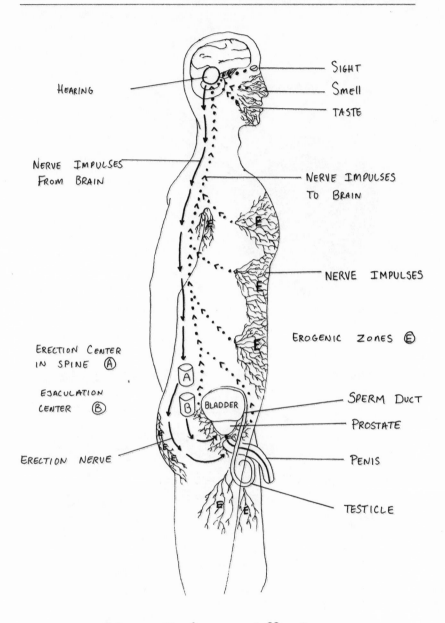

SIGHT
Smell
TASTE

HEARING

NERVE IMPULSES FROM BRAIN

NERVE IMPULSES TO BRAIN

NERVE IMPULSES

EROGENIC ZONES Ⓔ

ERECTION CENTER IN SPINE Ⓐ

EJACULATION CENTER Ⓑ

BLADDER

SPERM DUCT

PROSTATE

ERECTION NERVE

PENIS

TESTICLE

Nerve Pathways Affecting Stimulation of Erection and Ejaculation

References

1. Graedon, J. and T. *The People's Pharmacy 2.* (New York: Avon, 1980), 149-152.

2. Cohen, S. "Cannabis and Sex: Multifaceted Paradoxes." *Journal of Psychoactive Drugs.* 14:1-2 (Jan., 1982), 55-58.

3. Graedon, J. and T. *op. cit.*

4. Flatto, E. "Nutrition and Health Review." #46 *The Consumer's Medical Journal* (Spring, 1988), 11.

5. Kent, S. "Drugs to Boost Sexual Potency." *Geriatrics.* 36:7 (July 1981), 159-161.

6. *Physician's Desk Reference.* (Oradell, NJ: Edward R. Barnhart, 1990), 1123.

7. Morales, A. et al. *New England Journal of Medicine.* (Nov 12, 1981), 1221.

8. Goodman, G. *The Pharmacological Basis of Therapeutics,* 6th edition. (New York: Macmillan, 1988), 176-188.

9. *Medical World News.* (May 26, 1986), 82-83.

10. Ami Sidi, A. "Vasoactive Intracavernous Pharmacotherapy." *Urologic Clinics of North America.* 15:1 (Feb 1988), 98.

Chapter 4

Potency Devices and Surgeries

T O BE DEPRIVED OF THE ABILITY TO ACCOMPLISH normal sexual intercourse can be physically and psychologically devastating to many men. As recently as 1979, many physicians believed that over 90% of impotence was due to psychogenic causes. Since that time, new physical tests have demonstrated that over 50% of impotence has physical causes. As explained before, some pathological conditions that cause impotence are:

Diabetes mellitus

High blood pressure

Arteriosclerosis

Certain drugs and alcohol

Smoking

Multiple sclerosis

Liver or kidney damage

Parkinson's disease

Surgery or injury in the pelvic area

Spinal cord and brain injuries

Peyronie's disease

Priapism

These conditions typically affect either blood flow, hormone levels, or nerve impulses to the penis, all of which are vital to normal sexual functioning. Impotence can also be caused by a combination of physical and pyschogenic problems. It is important to determine the exact cause in each case before the problem can be treated successfully.

I am hopeful that information you have gleaned from previous chapters of this book will help correct any problem you may have with achieving and maintaining an erection. However, I strongly believe that anyone who suffers from erectile dysfunction should be informed on all viable methods of treatment available.

Mechanical Devices

Mechanical aids to allow sufficient penile rigidity for intercourse include externally positioned splints, suction/constriction devices, and penile implants. Two devices currently on the market are the Synergist Erection System and the Osbon Erec-Aid. The Erection System uses suction to draw the penis into a condom-shaped device that stays on the penis during intercourse.

The Erec-Aid uses suction to increase arterial blood flow. A hollow cylinder is placed around the penis and suction is applied. Once an erection has been achieved, the cylinder is removed and a constricting band is left in place. The success of this device depends on adequate blood flow, so it may not be appropriate for those with arterial insufficiency.[1]

Vacuum Erection Device (VED) is designed to produce an erection-like state, and makes the penis hard enough to penetrate the vagina and have sexual intercourse. It is intended for use by men who are impotent. The VED creates a vacuum which traps blood in the penis, making it hard. Constricting bands are then placed around the base of the penis to keep blood there and keep the penis hard after the vacuum is released. The bands may be safely left in place for up to thirty minutes by most men, the manufacturer states. The VED is not to be used before evaluation by a physician, and misuse of this product could result in swelling of the penis and/or serious injury to the penis including priapism, necrosis, and gangrene.

I advise against use of a rubber band around the base of the penis for constriction. The rubber band acts like a tourniquet and can actually cause gangrene to set in if left on too long.

Penile Implants

While penile implants have been used since 1960, they were not considered successful until Dr. Scott developed the first inflatable penile prosthesis in 1973. Two years later, Drs. Small and Carrion implanted semi-rigid rods made of silicone in the corpus cavernosa. Both of these devices proved relatively successful, and many of the present-day prosthetic implants are revised versions of the first implants.

A penile implant is a device that is surgically inserted within each of two spongy chambers (corpus cavernosa) of the penis, allowing an individual to have and maintain an erection when desired.

Rod implants consist of semi-rigid and malleable types. Although all rod implants create a permanent erection, some semi-rigid devices are hinged for concealability in clothing. Malleable implants (implants with an inner wire core) are bendable for concealment as well. Depending on implant use, there are varying degrees of concealability, functionality and dependability.

Inflatable implants consist of self-contained and multi-component types. Inflatable implants offer a more natural cosmetic result than rod implants and are becoming the preferred choice by men desiring penile implantation. The surgical procedure, similar to rod surgery, allows the implant to be placed within the penis using a small incision.

Am I a good candidate for an implant?

In *Love and Sex After 60*, Dr. Robert N. Butler and Myrna I. Lewis recommend guidelines which will help a man and his doctor reach a decision about the desirability of a penile implant. Not considered good candidates for penile prosthesis are men with:

- Untreated acute and severe depression. The depression should be successfully treated first.

- Serious psychosis or brain disease.

- Severe personality disorders, including the chronically dissatisfied.

- Severe and complicated marital problems.

- Impotence that is not clearly organic.

- Health conditions that contraindicate elective surgery.

A penile implant may be advisable when:

- It is clear that the impotence is primarily a chronic organic problem (caused, for example, by diabetes, vascular disease, problems associated with rectal or prostate surgery, pelvic nerve injury, or spinal cord injury).

- Sexual desire is strong and intercourse is greatly valued by both partners.

- There is evidence of continuing sexual activity between partners even in the absence of sexual intercourse.

- Presence of impotence per se is having a destructive effect on the relationship.

- Couple have a realistic understanding of what may be achieved, and both approve of the surgery.

Which one is right for me?

Discuss with your urologist the best penile implant for your particular needs. Implant cost, insurance coverage, activity of daily living, life-style and manual dexterity, to mention a few, are all factors to be considered in implant selection. Discuss with your physician specific differences of implant types, potential for breakage, and/or additional surgery, if required. Discuss implant warranty differences since the life expectancy of any mechanical device is unpredictable.

Most penile implants are made of medical grade silicone rubber. Although rejection may occur, silicone has been widely used in the medical field for over twenty years and is used for testicular implants as well.

Do not have unrealistic expectations. A penile implant allows a man to have an erect penis, but it is not able to make the penis appear or function as it did prior to the onset of impotence. Some loss of penile length, girth, or both may occur after surgery because the natural penis expands far better with normal blood flow than with a penile implant. The cosmetic results with inflatable implants normally improve with time due to improved tissue healing following surgery.

Penile implantation will not increase or decrease a man's sexual desire or harm ability to have an orgasm. Sperm production and ability to ejaculate should remain unaffected if present prior to onset of impotence. If you are uncircumcised, it may be necessary for your surgeon to remove the foreskin during the surgical procedure. General, local, or regional anesthesia may be used, depending on type of implant selected, surgical technique, and your overall physical condition.

Your partner should be involved in the decision process whenever possible. Most physicians encourage partners to become involved at the early stage of evaluation and testing so she may express her feelings and concerns. Most women are relieved to know that some form of treatment can be used when impotence cannot be corrected by any other means.

Immediately following surgery, you will experience some pain and discomfort which will subside within a few weeks. Medication might be prescribed to help ease discomfort. Your urologist will advise you when you may resume intercourse, which is normally four to six weeks following surgery.

When first resuming sexual intercourse, some couples may experience uncomfortable penetration. Uncomfortable intercourse occurs when there is a long absence of sexual activity. A change in sexual position or use of a lubricant may help alleviate uncomfortable penetration.

Rod Implants

The Surgitek Flexirod II semi-rigid implant is designed to conform to anatomy of the penis. A flexible hinge feature allows the penis to bend naturally, avoiding embarrassing clothing bulges. Manufacturer states that the Flexirod has been bent in the laboratory over fifteen million times without breakage. Malleable rods are designed with a stainless steel or silver wire core surrounded by silicone; the wire allows for positioning penis up or down.

The Dacomed DuraPhase positionable penile prosthesis is a pair of cylinders that provide penile rigidity. Manufacturer claims superior concealability, ease of operation and position-ability, eliminating the "springback" sometimes associated with malleable prostheses. It allows a man to position the device up for intercourse or down for concealment.

The Dacomed OmniPhase penile prosthesis is a pair of mechanically operated cylinders that produce rigidity or flac-cidity when activated or deactivated. When activated, the switch shortens the cable, bringing segments together to pro-duce rigidity. When deactivated, the cable lengthens to allow the segments to separate slightly, producing flaccidity. The simple activation mechanism provides patients with ability to gain rigidity or flaccidity with one simple motion.

Inflatables

The Surgitek Uniflate 1000 combines the pump and reservoir into one component, reducing the number of parts. It closely resembles a natural erection and is activated by squeez-ing the bulb implanted in the scrotum; an erection is created by squeezing the scrotal pump, causing fluid in the reservoir to flow into the penile cylinders implanted in the penile shaft. Returning the penis to a relaxed state is accomplished by squeezing a release ring located just above the bulb.

Other Surgeries

Other surgeries besides prosthetic insertion are now being performed for impotency. Angioplasty is done by passing a balloon through the clogged internal iliac or pudendal arteries. The balloon is then expanded to open up the artery and allow blood to pass into the corpora cavernosa of the penis. However, these dilations only appear to last for less than a year.

When ability to achieve erection is diminished because of poor blood flow from "hardening of the arteries" of arteriosclerosis, microvascular bypass surgery is done by attaching the nearby epigastric artery to the dorsal or cavernous arteries of the penis to bring blood in past the point of occlusion.[3,4]

While I could fill the book with prosthetic and other potency devices, I strongly believe that impotency is preventable, and correctable, by changing one's living habits for the better.

Take the case of Arthur, a 68-year-old accountant and a disabled navy veteran of World War II. Arthur was receiving a disability pension of 10% because of a hearing loss in his right ear after serving on a battleship during a major shelling attack on a Japanese island stronghold. He was standing too close to the cannons, and the noise and concussion damaged his ear drum.

Arthur was also unable to achieve an erection for the past three years except on one occasion. Since Arthur was receiving a disability pension that was service-connected, he was eligible for a penile implant.

Arthur consulted me about three weeks before the operation was scheduled. Arthur was, by our conventional standards, considered "successful"—and he wore the badges of success—ulcers and a pot belly. He also had arthritis, hay fever, asthma, sinus trouble, varicose veins, "smoker's cough" (chronic bronchitis), and arteriosclerosis. His serum cholesterol was 290 and his triglycerides 176—both extremely high. He took tranquilizers along to the office every morning and drank up to six cups of coffee daily. He had a reputation of having the disposition of a scorched wildcat. But he was considered a "success" in all except the most important aspect of living.

I finally convinced Arthur to postpone the operation, go on a zero-cholesterol program, stop smoking, and try to keep the coffee to no more than one cup a day. It was an extremely difficult ordeal, as well as a tremendous challenge for Arthur. But I confess to feeling a small share in his final victory.

A few months after Arthur started the program, he burst into my office with unbounded enthusiasm. "I had sex four times this week, for the first time in years, and I feel terrific!" he blurted out. His cholesterol and triglycerides had dropped to within normal parameters, and all his other medical problems showed marked improvement. Of course, the operation was unneeded and therefore canceled.

Arthur's case is not unique. Many others have avoided often painful penile operations with their uncertain results by simply changing their life-styles and getting rid of their bad habits.

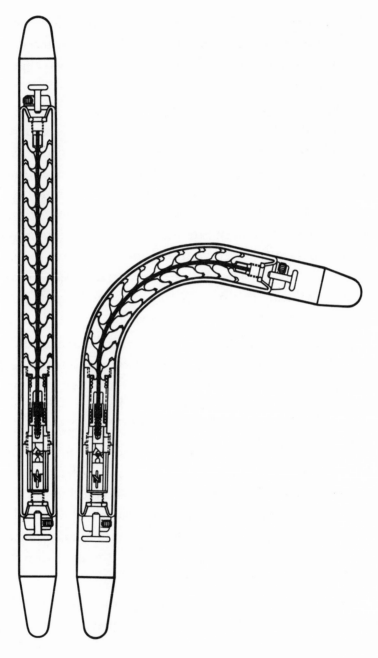

Omni-Phase Penile Prosthesis

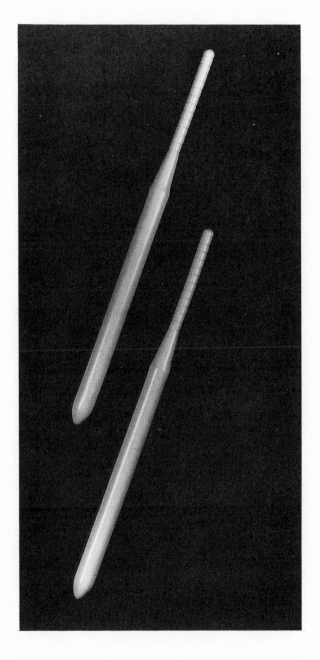

Surgitek

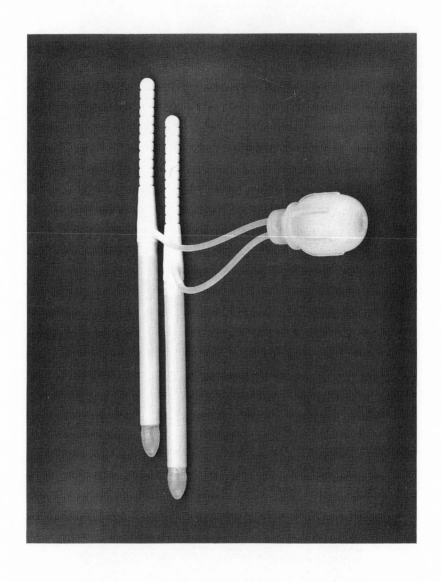

Uniflate® 1000 Inflatable Penile Implant

References

1. Mulligan, T., and P.G. Katz. "Erectile Failure in the Aged." *Journal of the American Geriatric Society.* 36:1 (Jan 1988), 59.

2. Butler, R.N., and M.I. Lewis. *Love and Sex After 60.* (New York: Harper and Row, 1988), 54.

3. Melman, A. "Evaluation and Management of Erectile Dysfunction." *Surgical Clinics of North America.* 68:5 (Oct 1988), 965-980.

4. Goldstein, I. "Overview of Types and Results of Vascular Surgical Procedures for Impotence." *CardioVascular and Interventional Radiology.* 11:4 (Aug 1988), 240-244.

Chapter 5

Premature Ejaculation and How to Cure It

A S A PHYSICIAN, LECTURER, AND SYNDICATED columnist for over twenty-five years, one of the most common sexual problems that is presented to me from men of all ages is the frustrating experience of premature ejaculation.

Premature ejaculation (PE) is defined in the *American Medical Association Family Medical Guide* as "orgasm in the man immediately after, or even before, the penis penetrates the woman's vagina in sexual intercourse."[1]

It is difficult to define premature ejaculation exactly, except in cases when ejaculation takes place before insertion of the penis into the vagina, because there are no sharp lines of distinction between "normal" and "abnormal" sexual behavior. While it may be difficult to set a definite "normal" time limit in intercourse before ejaculation, I believe the crucial balance between prematurity and normality lies in the absence of feeling in control over the ejaculatory reflex in the premature ejaculator.

Premature ejaculation is very rarely of organic origin, although conditions that cause irritation during sexual response, such as urethritis or prostatitis, may be contributing factors.

Ejaculation of seminal fluid during sexual intercourse is generally considered to be an involuntary reflex action, although it can be brought under voluntary control. Through proper training and self-discipline, ejaculation and orgasm in the male can be controlled for much longer periods of time.

Seminal emission is expulsion of secreted fluids from the prostate, seminal vesicles and testicles through the vasa deferentia into the urethra. Just before seminal emission occurs, the proximal end of the urethra closes by contraction of the internal bladder sphincter to prevent retrograde ejaculation into the bladder. Seminal emissions are initiated by sympathetic nerve fibers passing from spinal cord segments.

Ejaculation is achieved by a contraction of muscles in the pelvic floor, which results in an expulsion of semen from the urethra. The bulbocavernous and ischiocavernous muscles as well as other muscles are stimulated by spinal nerves from the base of the vertebral column.

Both emission and ejaculation are reflexes that are brought about by stimulation of the penis. These reflexes can be intentionally stimulated, but stimulation should stop before they are no longer under voluntary control. Emission and ejaculation result in an evacuation of secretions that have to be replaced.

Most strict religious observers believe that the sexual act should be controlled and that seminal fluid should be conserved; that the fluid a man ejaculates during sexual relations contains the human seed, and to waste this fluid as a form of pleasure is a tremendous drain on the body's resources. Buddhism, Catholicism, Hinduism, Islam, Orthodox Judaism, and Protestantism all have sexual control as part of their tenets.

Aristotle, Plato, Moses, Buddha, Jesus, Mohammed, Mary Baker Eddy, Sigmund Freud, Yogi Ramacharaka, Gandhi, and Ellen G.H. White are some of the religious leaders and philosophers who believed in sexual control in one form or another.

However, sex for procreation only is generally unworkable for the vast majority. On the other hand, sexual control, in that the man withholds ejaculation, is entirely feasible and satisfying when no offspring are desired. Of course additional birth control methods should be used to prevent unwanted pregnancy.

There have been a number of methods and techniques for curing premature ejaculation and prolonging intercourse without ejaculating. Some of these methods include the use of condoms to make the penis less sensitive to sexual excitement, application of anesthetic ointments to the penis, or use of alcohol and sedative drugs to reduce sexual excitement. None has proved extirely satisfactory, and some are even harmful. They may reduce sensations of sexual pleasure, but usually do not improve a man's ejaculatory control once he has reached the peak of erotic arousal.

It should be axiomatic that the sex act in humans, like all other living creatures, was intended primarily for continuation of the species. But in humans it can and should also be an act of love and communion.

When a man ejaculates before or soon after entering the vagina, the sexual attempt is quite frustrating to both partners and can be as anxiety-producing as impotence itself. It can sometimes lead to temporary or even permanent impotence. It can also lead to hostility and other negative feelings between the couple.

For both partners to derive maximum pleasure, a man should be able to control ejaculation. One of the most gratifying acts in life is giving pleasure to someone you love. And one of the manifestations of love is putting someone else's pleasure before your own. Therefore, a man who truly loves a woman will want to put her pleasure and satisfaction first. And this applies especially during sexual intercourse.

Since the biological response of the average male is to ejaculate within two minutes after vaginal penetration[2], and since few women are able to reach orgasm within two minutes[3], most men must learn how to retard emission and ejaculation.

In order for ejaculation to be brought under voluntary control, a certain amount of self-discipline must be developed. *Self-discipline, self-control,* and *will power* all have the same connotation. They may all be defined as *mental muscle.* And like any other muscle, the more we use it, the stronger it becomes.

Acquiring self-discipline in controlling ejaculation is difficult at first. However, doing things that are difficult is good for you! It was difficult to send man to the moon, but we did it.

Difficult and *impossible* are not the same words! Some people think because something is difficult to attain, they shouldn't attempt it. However, after developing the habit of controlling ejaculation, you will find it becomes second nature.

In 1956, Dr. James Seamans, a urologist, introduced a technique for curing premature ejaculation. Dr. Seamans' premise was that the primary cause of premature ejaculation was a "rapid reflex mechanism" which prevented a man from gaining control of orgasm and ejaculation.

To remedy this disability, Dr. Seamans developed his method of prolonging the neuromuscular reflex of ejaculation. The method involves a manual stimulation of the man's penis by his partner until he feels he is about to experience orgasm. When he feels his climax is approaching, he motions his partner to stop. After several of these stroking sessions the man will ejaculate.

This technique should be repeated once or more a week for about a month or so, or until the man can tolerate the stimulation indefinitely without ejaculating. Dr. Seamans considered a patient cured once he reached this point. Of the patients in his initial experiments, he claimed a 100% cure rate within one month.

A variation of Seamans' method was used by Masters and Johnson with a reported 98% success rate. This method, called the "squeeze technique," is similar to Seamans' stroke technique except that when the man signals that he feels close to orgasm, the woman squeezes the penis just below the rim of the glans until the pain makes his erection subside. This stroking/squeezing procedure is repeated a number of times until control is attained.

I want to inject at this point that there is no biological need to ejaculate the seminal fluid. If a man doesn't urinate or defecate, he will die in a short period of time; both urine and excrement are toxic to the body if retained. But seminal fluid is not a waste product that must be regularly eliminated like urine. There is no disease or physiological harm caused by not releasing semen. On the contrary, seminal fluid contains hormones that are important to our harmonious development.

When men overexpend this vital fluid, secretions of the sexual glands and hormones are lost and the body is deprived of valuable substances, resulting in mental and physical weakness, inability to concentrate, and a less tenacious memory.[4]

In the event that you should lose control and ejaculate, do not dispair, but strengthen your resolve to master control the next time.

Once you have gained control and overcome any tendency to ejaculate prematurely, you are ready to take the next step and master the new sexual science of seminal conservation, described in the next chapter.

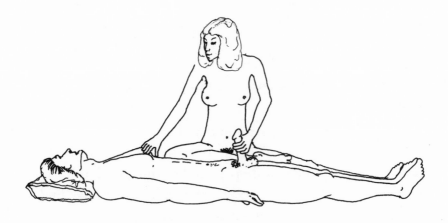

Seaman Method For Treatment
Of Premature Ejaculation

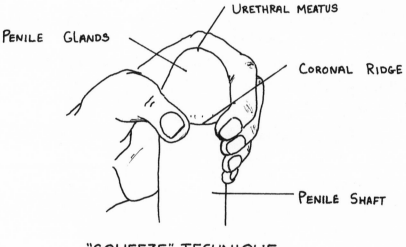

URETHRAL MEATUS

PENILE GLANDS

CORONAL RIDGE

PENILE SHAFT

"SQUEEZE" TECHNIQUE

"Squeeze" Technique

References

1. *American Medical Association Family Medical Guide.* (New York: Random House, 1982), 614.

2. *Merck Manual,* 13th edition. (Rahway, NJ: Merck, Sharp and Dohme, 1977) 1772.

3. Ibid, 1773.

4. Flatto, Edwin, *Look Younger, Think Clearer, Live Longer.* (Miami: Plymouth Books, 1977), 23.

Chapter 6

The New Science of Seminal Conservation

THIS NEW SCIENCE IS BASED UPON THOUSANDS of years of study, observation, and experimentation. It has been refined and developed to a new degree, thus entitling it to the appellation "new." The science of seminal conservation allows you to conserve seminal fluid for nourishing, improving and perfecting the body and brain when reproduction is not mutually desired.

Nature puts the most valuable ingredients in the seed in all forms of life in order to provide for continuation of the species. And the fluid (semen) a man discharges during sexual relations contains the human seed.

The human seed, of course, contains all essential elements necessary to create another human being when it is united with an ovum. It contains forces capable of creating life! Doesn't common sense decree that such a vital fluid be carefully conserved, rather than thoughtlessly squandered? How can a state of health, energy and power be built when the most basic elements are being excessively squandered?

The seminal fluid is a viscid, proteinaceous fluid composed of secretory products of the testes, epididymis, seminal vesicles, prostate gland, and Cowper's gland. It is rich in

149

potassium, iron, lecithin, vitamin E, protease, spermine, albumen, phosphorus, calcium and other organic minerals and vitamins.

The average normal ejaculation, about two to five cubic centimeters of semen, contains 200 to 500 million sperm which are rich in nuclear proteins, the male hormones or androgens such as testosterone, and other essential elements. The Sertoli cells in the testes produce another hormone, Inhibin.

These hormones, or androgens, including testosterone, go directly into the bloodstream if not ejaculated and are carried to every part of the body. They stimulate the pituitary gland and creative centers of the brain.

Each one of these millions of sperm carry 23 chromosomes, split chromosomes, prostaglandins, genes, bioelectricity, and all vitamins, enzymes and minerals necessary for the creation of another human being when united with an ovum.

An analysis of both brain cells and semen shows great similarities. Both are very high in phosphorus, sodium, magnesium and chlorine. The sex glands and brain cells are intimately connected physiologically, but are adversaries in the sense that they are both competing for the same nutritional elements from the identical bloodstream. In this sense, the brain and the sexual organs are also competitors in using bodily energy and nutrition.

There are only so many nutrients in the bloodstream. The body can only assimilate limited quantities of nutrients in a given period of time. Phosphorus, for example, is required in both the thinking and reproductive processes. Still, the body can only assimilate finite or limited quantities of phosphorus from the diet to meet these demands in a twenty-four hour period. If most nutrients in the blood are going into meeting demands of the gonads, and being ejaculated, there will be little left over to meet nutritional demands of the rest of the body and brain.

The energy of the body is most potent when used in one direction. An analogy: if you were to open the spigot in your kitchen sink while all other faucets were shut, you'd have great water pressure from that faucet; but if you simultaneously flush the toilet, turn on the shower, water the lawn, fill the bath tub and run the washer, the water pressure at each outlet would drop dramatically. The same is true of the body. A man cannot think or perform his best when much of his energy and blood's nutriments are expended in the discharge of semen.

Most sexual relationships begin with a great deal of sexual activity during which the male ejaculates frequently. He just can't seem to get enough. After each ejaculation he becomes more depleted and exhausted. The loss of energy due to excessive ejaculation is a slow and subtle process that most men don't usually notice until it's too late. After countless episodes, a deterioration of the body sets in. As a man gets older, he may rationalize his lack of energy and loss of sexual vigor on his age. He is only too happy to continue pumping out his semen, sometimes even *paying* for the privilege, and accelerating the deterioration.

One of my most vivid cases involved a successful attorney, 42 years of age, a former football player on his college team. What I saw was a mere shadow of his former well-built body. He looked closer to 60 than 42. His body and face sagged and he walked and moved like a man of 70. His family was convinced he had some serious disease. He seemed to have hit rock bottom. I took his case history and finally inquired into his sexual routine. He casually confessed that he indulged in fellatio (oral sex) "with a beautiful prostitute who visits my office every afternoon."

Several days later I had occasion to visit his office in the afternoon and immediately recognized the woman in his reception room from his description. She was a tall, statuesque brunette with broad shoulders, about 35, almost Amazonian in build and appearance. The attorney came out and introduced us. She was friendly and quite talkative, an asset, no doubt, for attracting new clients. During our conversation she mentioned that she was a vegetarian, which was of interest to me since I am a vegetarian also.

"What do you eat for protein?" she inquired.

"Nuts, seeds and vegetables," I replied. "And what do you eat for your protein?"

"Seminal fluid," she replied, unashamedly frank. "It's a complete protein and has all the best elements and vitamins needed to nourish my body!"

I looked her over again carefully from top to bottom and couldn't help but agree that her dietary habits were certainly producing a beautiful specimen of womanhood. Then I thought of my unfortunate patient, the brilliant attorney, who was sacrificing his health and strength for a few moments of sensualism and, to add insult to injury, was *paying* for the privilege.

Afterward I explained to the attorney what this drain on his vital fluid was doing to him and how he could enjoy normal sex without wasting his life force. He came to see me eight months later and I could scarcely recognize him. He appeared years younger, he bounded up the steps three at a time, and his face reflected a picture of health and vitality. He told me how he enjoyed sexual intercourse up to five times a day, never losing a drop of his vital fluid, and had stiff erections instead of rubbery, soft ones.

I want to reassert at this point that vigorous health is the best aphrodisiac. And an important factor in obtaining vigorous health is the fuller knowledge of nutrition in meeting the demands of an active sexual, fulfilling life. Not only can a proper diet and these gentle exercises keep your arteries clean so blood can flow freely to all your vital organs as well as your corpora cavernosa penis, but they can also replenish the power of every cell in your body.

Cooked, canned, fried, processed, irradiated, barbecued, microwaved, degerminated, preserved, chemicalized, homogenized, pasteurized and otherwise devitalized foods are not the best materials to be converted into healthy tissues, blood and vital organs needed for vigorous health—and certainly not to meet the demands of an active sexual life. Poor health and/or poor diet demand that a man ejaculate no more than once a month if he wants to avoid mental and physical bankruptcy.

Can you have an orgasm without ejaculating? Some experts think so. Note the following from *Male Sexuality*:

"Most authorities have accepted the contention of Masters and Johnson that while women have several different patterns of orgasmic response, only one type of ejaculatory response is possible for men. We disagree with this thinking, having ourselves experienced different ejaculatory patterns and having heard from a number of other men that they sometimes have ejaculations substantially different from the Masters and Johnson standard. Sometimes the excitement is so intense before ejaculation that it in itself feels like a long orgasm, and the actual ejaculation not only doesn't add anything to it but is experienced as a letdown."

"While ejaculation and orgasm are often used synonymously even by some sex experts, we find it useful to distinguish between them. Ejaculation is the physical process involved in propelling the semen through the penis. Orgasm refers to what you feel. Generally the two go together; you ejaculate and enjoy very pleasurable feelings. But one can occur without the other. You can have orgasms without ejaculating. Some men have trained themselves to do this and, according to their reports, have been able to have multiple orgasms like women.

"And some men, who have trained themselves carefully to tune into their sensations during sex, say that they sometimes notice very high peaks of feeling long before ejaculation. Were they not so indoctrinated in the idea that orgasm occurs only with pelvic contractions and ejaculations, they would be inclined to call these peaks orgasms."

The idea of conserving the seminal fluid is not a new one. The Bible has many references to the harmfulness of wasting this vital fluid. In the allegory of Samson and Delilah, for example, it seems quite obvious that the beautiful but cunning Delilah knew that the secret of Samson's strength resided in his seminal fluid. When she went to bed with Samson, she was out to drain him of his vital fluid, not shear him of his long hair. She was sophisticated enough to know that if she emptied him of his seminal fluid, his strength would diminish. After Samson practiced a period of abstinence, he regained his strength, and he was able to break his chains, bringing down the supporting pillars where he was held captive and thereby destroying himself, his prison and his captors.

Onan's sin of casting his seed upon the ground (for which his penalty was death) is another Biblical warning against wasting seminal fluid. Apparently the sages who wrote the Bible realized the biological power of seminal fluid and the wisdom of conserving it for purposes higher than just momentary sensual self-indulgence. One purpose of circumcision is to desensitize the glans penis so sexual desire is more easily controlled. It is said that Abraham, the first Jew, was circumcised to remind himself of his covenant with God.

Next to the Bible, probably the oldest sex instruction book was the S'u Wen Ne' I Ching, written over forty centuries ago. For several centuries it was studied and practiced by Chinese nobility, but for some unknown reason it was suppressed. However, many of its teachings were recorded and still practiced by followers of Taoism. They believed that retaining the seminal fluid contributed to health, vitality and long life.

According to Taoist historians, it was considered the duty of a member of the nobility to satisfy at least seven of his wives or concubines daily. To accomplish this, a method of sexual intercourse was developed by which he could retain his ejaculation so that his health and vitality were not drained.

The Taoists finally developed this method of "injaculating", or having an orgasm without ejaculating. This was accomplished by pressing an acupuncture point midway between the scrotum and anus (perineum) in the male just before ejaculation was anticipated so that the ejaculate was prevented from leaving the body during orgasm. Thus the semen was recycled and reabsorbed into his bloodstream.

If you would like to learn more about this method of lovemaking and are willing to devote considerable study time and effort, I suggest the following reading: *The Tao of Sexology* by

Dr. Stephen T. Chang, *The Tao of Love and Sex: The Ancient Chinese Way to Ecstasy* by John Chang, and *Taoist's Secrets of Love: Cultivating Male Sexual Energy* by Mantak Chia.[3]

In athletics, most professional coaches and trainers forbid sexual relations before a contest to conserve contestants' energy and power. Prize fighters also observe strict sexual abstinence during training and before a bout. In his book, *Muhammed Ali—The Greatest,* Olympic boxing coach Harry Wiley says: "There's a kid just come down here named Cassius Clay. If you bet on him every time he fights, you'll be a rich man, 'cause he won't lose a single fight. I believe his thing is sexual control. And he's got it. Any kid who can control his sex can win the title. I believe it."

The Technique of Seminal Conservation

Before starting my seminal conservation method, the following exercises should be performed on a daily basis for several days to a week or more in order to develop muscles in the pelvic area:

Squeeze and relax gluteal muscles (in the buttocks) fifty times in the morning and fifty times before retiring at night. (Also good to avoid prostate trouble.)

Shoulder stand. (See page 166.)

I have found the following technique to be highly successful in not only conserving seminal fluid indefinitely when children are not desired, but to promote harmonious marital relations as well. I am proud to state that I have numerous letters in my files attesting to the benefits of this method.

Here is my method of seminal conservation:

The usual foreplay is engaged in by both partners with mutual kissing and caressing of the breasts and all other erogenous parts of each others' bodies as desired, leaving stimulation of the female genitalia for last.

The foreplay should not be hurried, and the male organ should not be permitted to enter the vagina deeply at this point, although the penis may be in close contact with the moist membrane of the female labia.

In the event that the labia is not sufficiently lubricated after a reasonable period of time has passed, a small amount of K-Y jelly or other lubricant should be introduced into the vagina to prevent excoriation.

While lying thus relaxed, the woman raises both her legs by bending her knees and pulling them upward toward her chest or assumes any other preferred position. The man gently parts the labia of the vagina and partially inserts his penis.

Deep penetration of the vagina is not advised at this point. But close contact between the penis and moist membrane of the *labia majora* or inner lips is important. There may be silent meditation or speaking of words of tenderness.

After several minutes, the male should take his organ and rub it against the clitoris a few times. Be sure the entire vaginal area is well lubricated, including the lips of the vulva (labia majora and minora) which enclose the clitoris.

Whatever position is assumed, do not plunge the entire length of the shaft of the penis full depth at this time. Just insert it about halfway at first, then remove it after about twenty seconds.

This may be very difficult at first. Resist the temptation. Rest a few moments. Insert your organ again—this time a little deeper. Tell your partner not to move at this time.

If at any time you should feel as though you are getting close to ejaculation, *hold your breath* and at the same time turn the tongue backwards as far as you can, pressing the tip of the tongue against the roof of your mouth.

It is important to hold your breath whenever you feel you may be approaching orgasm. There is a Hindu master who declares: "So long as the breath is in motion, the semen moves also. When breath ceases to move, the semen is likewise at rest."

If you still feel lack of control, you should withdraw your organ completely and rest it until you have it under control. Do not allow the ejaculate to enter the prostate or urethra, which is the *point-of-no-return* at any time. Anytime you feel you are getting too excited and in danger of losing control, hold your breath while doubling the tongue backwards as far as you can against the roof of your mouth.

Perhaps you will feel more confident at first by resting an hour or two and later resuming after you have gained more control. Remember to start all over from the beginning each time, and patience is definitely a virtue when it comes to making love. Also keep in mind that it takes practice to master control.

If at any time ejaculation should unintentionally occur, don't be discouraged; try another time.

The more you practice, the greater control you will develop. Men should do the exercises in this book, and women should practice squeezing the male organ when it is inside by contracting the vaginal and perineal muscles. Resist the temptation to move when your female partner requests you not to. Otherwise, too much stimulation at the wrong time will result in loss of control and reaching the point-of-no-return. Timing is very important.

It is in the first few minutes of the sex act when there is most sensitivity. If you control the act during these moments by not rushing, you will find that you can continue for a longer period of time without feeling the urge to ejaculate.

You can learn to control the length of the sex act and, if so desired, the frequency of the sex act, by not ejaculating, without harm, but with benefit systemically.

With each successive episode your control should improve. You should soon be able to have sexual intercourse as often as you desire, with no loss of power, energy, strength, vigor, potency and health, as long as you do not waste your seminal fluid.

Another of my cases involved a couple who very much wanted to have a child of their own. Jim was 61, a highly successful business executive; Kay was 37, and had never been pregnant before. The couple had been trying, without success, to conceive a child for twenty-five months prior to consulting me, although they had seen an infertility specialist who had prescribed fertility drugs to Kay.

Jim's medical history and my examination revealed he had arteriosclerosis, constipation, varicose veins, hemorrhoids, an enlarged prostate, and arthritis. His sperm count was low, his cholesterol level and blood pressure were very high, and he was a premature ejaculator whenever he was able to achieve an erection hard enough for coitus. When I spoke to Kay alone, she said that at times Jim had a "disposition like a scorched wild cat."

Jim described himself as "mostly vegetarian, eating only chicken, fish, dairy products and eggs, with an occasional Big Mac or cheeseburger with fries." He also "smoked a few cigars a week, had only two cups of coffee before lunch, and a few beers or a cocktail before or after dinner." He had no idea why his cholesterol and blood pressure were high, and he wanted to know what drugs I could give him to bring them down.

I then asked him to give me an idea of what he was accustomed to eating on a daily basis. This was his program:

Breakfast: Synthetic "orange" juice, two fried eggs with bacon strips or sausage *or* sugar coated "corn" flakes, two pats of butter on white toast, and one or two cups of coffee with whitener or cream.

Lunch: Fried chicken with barbecue sauce, French fries, pie and coffee.

Dinner: Canned soup, fish, canned peas, and mashed frozen potatoes, pie and coffee.

At midnight: Almost everything left in the refrigerator, plus coffee.

This "successful" man has "eaten" four times. But what has he *really* eaten for his health?

Nothing!

I agreed to accept their case on condition they would follow my "prescriptions," not 90% but 100%. Both agreed, and I explained that my "prescriptions" were not available in any drugstore but rather involved a complete change of attitude and living habits.

I immediately wrote out a dietary program similar to the ones in this book, started him on an exercise and walking program, and had them both eliminate coffee and smoking. I also gave them instructions on how to overcome Jim's premature ejaculation.

Eight months later I was informed that Kay was pregnant, and she eventually had a healthy baby girl; a year after that, she became pregnant again, this time giving birth to a boy.

One of the questions I am often asked is which coital position is best? Actually, a man who has mastered this science should be able to control his ejaculation in any position. However, the woman on top in the prone position should enable the man to have more control over his ejaculation. For this reason, it is a very good position for beginners.

The only problem with this position is that a man needs a good stiff erection in order to penetrate properly. A rubbery or semi-hard erection will not serve the purpose. To overcome this drawback for a man with a "semi," some couples start with the man on top and after penetration roll over so that the woman is on top.

Another memorable case involved a 71-year-old man, 5'10" tall, 260 pounds, who had recently married a woman of forty. His wife complained that he only wanted sex once or twice a month. She was in relatively good health. The man had a boggy and irritated prostate gland, didn't exercise, was over-weight, smoked five or six cigarettes daily, and his cholesterol level was 300. He was on medication to lower his hypertension.

I prescribed a zero-cholesterol dietary program and re-quested that he eliminate the cigarette habit, which he was able to do. I also put him on a walking program and had him perform at least five pelvic exercises daily, including contracting his buttocks and stopping and starting his urinary stream. I also counseled him on my technique of multiple daily inter-course. Eight months later his checkup revealed a normal prostate, his cholesterol was down to 200, his weight was down to 190 pounds, and his blood pressure was normal without medication. The most incredible part, however, was that he reported having "sexual congress" up to five times a day without ejaculating, and his wife was delighted!

Because training oneself to control sexual intercourse before reaching the point-of-no-return is difficult, most men are reluctant to try it. Almost all of the time and pleasure in sexual intercourse is derived during the pre-ejaculation phase. Learning to be satisfied at that point is crucial. Like they say on Wall Street: "The bulls make money and the bears make money but the hogs get slaughtered!"

The master of Taoist philosophy, Dr. Stephen T. Chang, wrote: "When the average male ejaculates, he loses about one tablespoon of semen. According to scientific research, the nutritional value of this amount of semen is equal to that of two pieces of New York steak, ten eggs, six oranges, and two lemons combined. That includes proteins, vitamins, minerals, amino acids, everything . . . Ejaculation is often called 'coming.' The precise word for it should be 'going,' because everything—the erection, vital energy, millions of live sperm, hormones, nutrients, even a little of the man's personality goes away. It is a great sacrifice for the man, spiritually, mentally, and physically."

To illustrate how much of a "ball" some older men are having by practicing seminal conservation, let me cite the case of Harry, who recently celebrated his 82nd birthday. Harry has a whole stable of women. Sex-starved women keep calling him from early morning to late at night. They compete, beg, bribe and cajole Harry to spend the night with them. They shower him with gifts, invite him to elegant parties, restaurants, even on cruises.

If you think Harry is a Clark Gable type, you are wrong. He is not by any standards what one would call good looking, dashing, or rich. Harry is bald, has a large black mole near the end of his nose, his false teeth drop and click whenever he opens his mouth, and he gives you a shower bath when he talks. His main income is his Social Security check.

What is the secret of Harry's popularity with all these women? Two things. He is able to perform sexually without ejaculating, and he likes women his own age. At age 82 there are at least four women for every man. And for every man 82 who can still perform sexually, four cannot.

That means there are sixteen sex-starved women available for every man at that age. Harry has learned to satisfy all these women because he has learned seminal conservation.

Remember, with a little patience and practice, the rewards of multiple daily intercourse can be yours!

The scientists of old have put great value upon the vital fluid and they have insisted upon its strong transmutation into the highest form of energy for the benefit of society.

Mahatma Gandhi

The strength of the body, the light of the eyes, the entire life of the man is slowly being lost by too much loss of vital fluid.

Jewish Code of Laws
Sec. Orach Chaim;
Ch. 240; Parag. 14

The stuff of the sexual life is the stuff of art; if it is expended in one channel it is lost for the others.

Havelock Ellis

Leg Lift Exercise

Lying on back, raise the legs alternately one at a time to perpendicular. Keep knee of the raised leg straight and toes pointed. Hold for 30 seconds and then lower to floor. Now raise both legs in same movement and continue as long as comfortable.

You may also practice this exercise on a slant board, keeping the feet higher than the body. Also for correcting and preventing intestinal hernia.

Sex Exercises

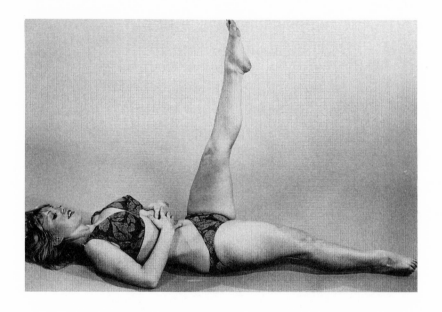

Sex Exercises - Leg Lift Exercise

"Shoulder Stand"

Lying on back, raise trunk to approximately 90 degree angle with arms supporting hips as shown. Hold this position as long as comfortable. Lower spine gently to floor. Do this exercise whenever you have need and time.

Also beneficial for varicose veins.

Sex Exercises

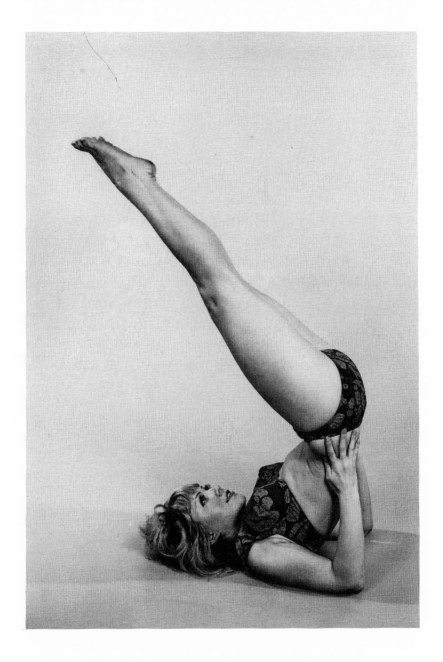

Sex Exercises - Shoulder Stand

"Flutter Kick"

Lying on slant board with legs raised, as shown, kick from the hips as though you were swimming. When you are tired, remain resting on the slant board with the feet elevated. Elevating the feet allows the blood in the legs to return to the heart by gravity rather than pressure. After resting, do another set if comfortable. Also, especially for preventing and correcting intestinal hernia.

Sex Exercises

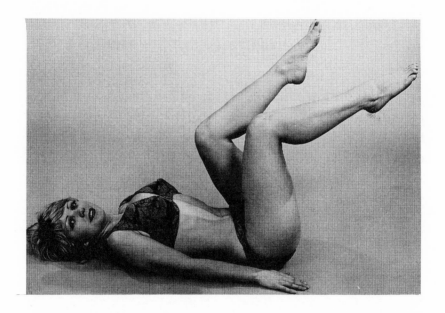

Sex Exercises - "Flutter Kick"

"Head Stand"

Using the low parallel bars is a good alternative to standing on the head since it avoids pressure to the cranium and is easier to do. This exercise allows gravity to assist in the return of blood to the heart. An assistant should be available for beginners.

Sex Exercises

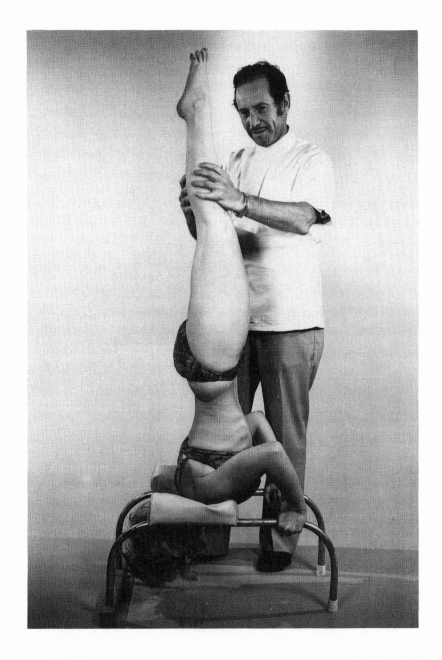

Sex Exercises - "Head Stand"

Bicycle Ride Exercise

Using the slant board, with head lower than feet, assume the inverted position holding sides of board for balance. Now take a long "bicycle ride" cycling as rapidly as possible at times but stop before you become over-tired.

This exercise is also beneficial for the prevention and correction of most cases of intestinal hernia.

Sex Exercises

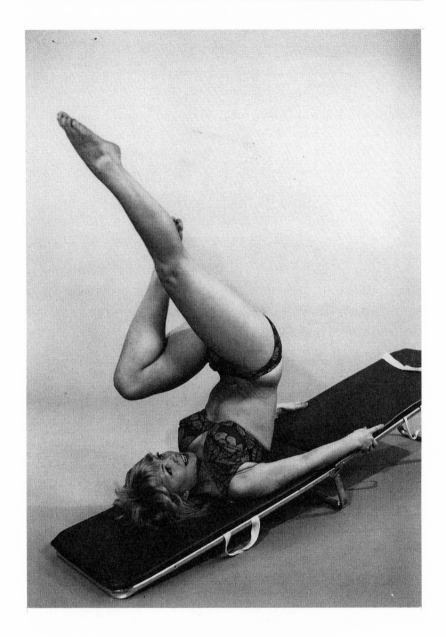

Sex Exercise - Bicycle Ride
Exercise

Slant Board Isometrics

Lying on back with head lower than feet on slant board, slowly raise both legs about 14 inches from the board. Now spread apart. (If assistant is available, have her give resistance while you are trying to spread them apart.)

Another variation of this exercise is to try to raise the legs while the assistant pushed them down. This exercise is also beneficial for arthritis, especially if the hips and legs are involved.

Sex Exercises

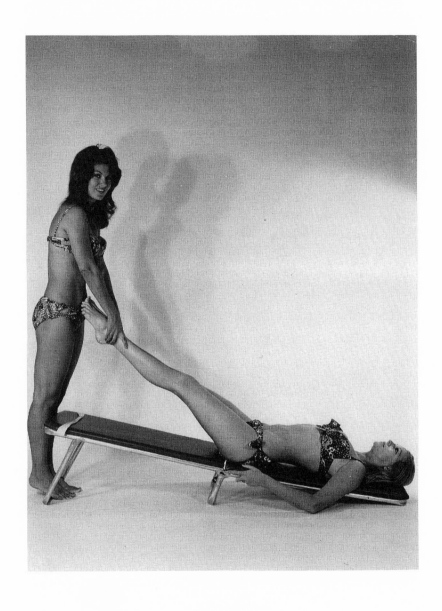

Sex Exercises - Slant Board
Isometrics

References

1. Zilbergeld, B. *Male Sexuality.* (New York: Bantam, 1978), 126-127.

2. Ali, Muhammed. *Muhammed Ali—The Greatest.* (New York: Random House, 1975), 130.

3. Chang, Stephen T. *The Tao of Sexology.* (San Francisco: Tao Publishing, 1988)

Chapter 7

How to Increase the Pleasure Women Can Give and Get From You

ONE OF THE GREAT MODERN TRAGEDIES resulting from lack of proper exercise is loss of sensation in the vagina during sexual relations resulting from stretching of perineal and vaginal muscles during childbirth.

In the process of childbirth, vaginal walls and muscles may be stretched as much as a foot in order to permit the baby's entire body to pass through. A woman who gives birth in an unconscious and drugged state, who fails to nurse her baby, and above all, who neglects exercises to restore the pelvic and perineal muscles to their normal prepartum positions may find that both she and her husband have to pay a very steep price when they lose much of the control and pleasurable sensation normally experienced during sexual intercourse.

Nature did not envision a woman missing the greatest emotional experience of her life in a state of unconsciousness, or having her legs up in stirrups during childbirth.

Neither did nature plan for the cow to become foster mother to the human race. There is a physiological connection between the breasts and the vaginal muscles. The woman who nurses her child is not only at less risk to get cancer of the breast and uterus, but each time her baby nurses from her breast, her vaginal muscles contract, helping restore them to their normal prepartum position.

Most women who give birth in a drugged and unconscious state find that their vaginal muscles have become so flaccid that neither they nor their mate feels much sensation during sexual relations.

Nature is very efficient. Our creator designed the perineal muscles in the woman's vagina to contract on the male's penis in order to milk remaining seminal fluid from the urethra to prevent the waste of any remaining drops.

In addition to preventing waste, nature has also provided that this vaginal constriction be an extremely pleasurable sensation to both partners in order to provide incentive for continuation of the species.

Much pleasurable sensation and communion is lost when the vaginal muscles are flaccid and can no longer perform functionally.

The exercises which follow, aimed at restoring muscular control to the female genitals, are to preserve and enhance human pleasure and happiness and to increase the efficiency of copulation as nature intended.

Leg Raising Exercise

Holding on to chair with left hand for support, raise right leg sideways as high as comfortable.

Restores control to the pelvic and genital musculature. Also for preventing varicose veins and disorders of the lower digestive tract.

Sex Exercises

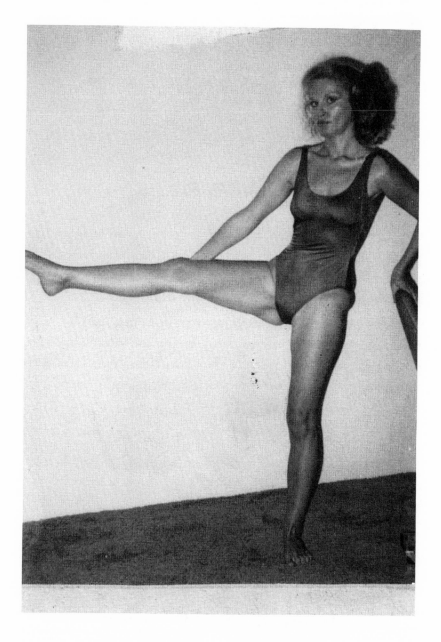

Sex Exercises - Leg Raising
Exercise

Leg Raising Execise

Lying on abdomen, both legs together, arms at sides, fists pressing against floor or hard mattress. Keeping knees stiff, slowly raise legs several inches off floor—then hold for several seconds, and then slowly lower to the floor again.

You may repeat this exercise if comfortable. This is one of the most important exercises for restoring the internal muscles of the vagina and abdomen to their prepartum positions. Also for strengthening the lower back muscles, and to correct backache, hemorrhoids, and disorders of the lower intestinal tract.

Increased Sexual Efficiency

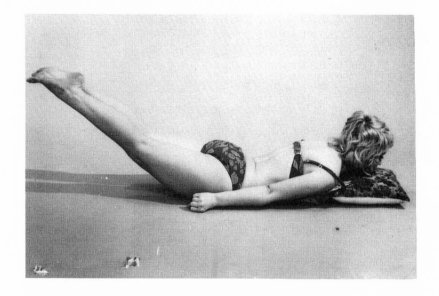

Increased Sexual Efficiency - Leg
Raising Exercise

Kneeling Exercise

Kneeling with palms flat on floor, bring right leg as far forward and at as much of a right angle to the body as possible. Hold for several seconds and then return to kneeling position. Alternate with other leg. Repeat.

This exercise strengthens the pelvic muscles and restores order to the abdominal and vaginal zone. Also for constipation and intestinal disorders.

Increased Sexual Efficiency

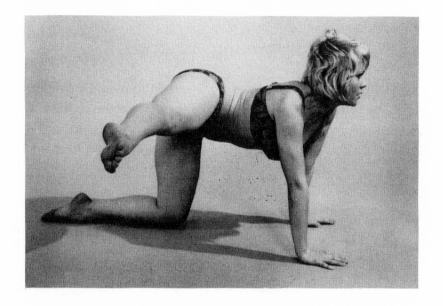

Kneeling Exercise - Increased
Sexual Efficiency

"Swimming" Exercise

Lying on stomach, keeping knees straight, kick the legs from the hips as though you were swimming. For strengthening abdominal and vaginal muscles. Also for varicose veins, disorders of the lower intestinal tract, hemorrhoids, and constipation.

Increased Sexual Efficiency

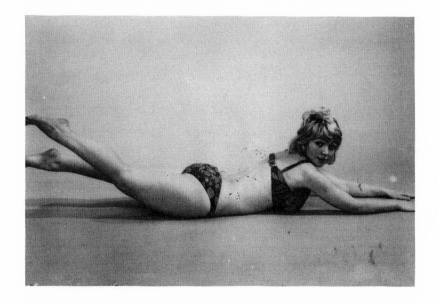

Increased Sexual Efficiency -
"Swimming" Exercise

Leg Exercises

Lying on left side, bring right leg as far forward as possible. Now bring it all the way to the rear. Now turn over and do the opposite side. Repeat if not tired.

Also for constipation and intestinal disorders.

Increased Sexual Efficiency

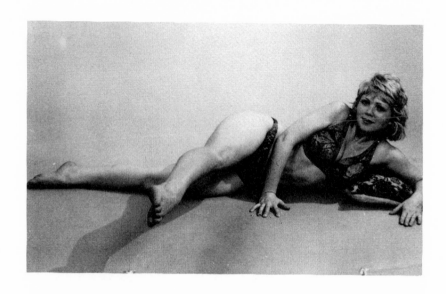

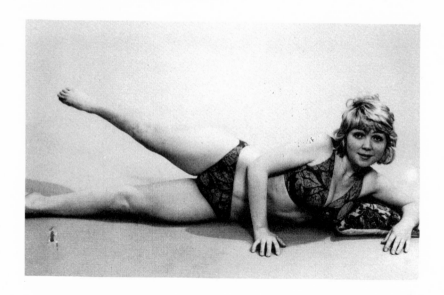

Increased Sexual Efficiency - Leg
Exercises

Chapter 8

How to Think Yourself Potent

OPTIMISM, HAPPINESS, JOY, AND A GOOD sense of humor are all vitally important to a man's healthy sexual functioning. Depression, fear, jealousy, guilt and resentment can all be far worse than anything else in ruining a man's ability to get and sustain an erection. Illness and/or pain can also destroy potency.

For example, if a man is suffering from hemorrhoids and his mind is dwelling on his painful and itching rectum, it is going to be extremely difficult for him to maintain an erection. Our brain cannot concentrate on two different things at the same time. We may think we have this ability, but our mind is actually darting back and forth, unable to aim its full attention to either, and therefore unable to direct a full blood supply to both at the same time.

Sometimes a careless or disparaging remark can devastate a person. When that happens, say to yourself, "An intelligent person cannot insult me, and no intelligent person would!"

One of the first signs of what can be a serious mental illness is this: a loss of interest. Because to be well-adjusted means that you *are* interested. Interested in others, interested in sharing with others, being with others. Interested in yourself and *interacting* with others.

A minister had just finished delivering an inspiring sermon on a Sunday morning. One of his parishoners came back and said, "That was a damn good talk you delivered this morning, Reverend!"

"What did you say?"

"I said that was a damn good talk you delivered this morning."

"Don't you think those are strong words to be using in church?"

"Well, Reverend, I thought it was such a fine talk that I put a hundred dollar bill in the collection plate!"

"Oh, thank you very much," replied the Reverend. "It takes a hell of a lot of money to run a church!"

A man was once asked what he thought of indifference and apathy. "I don't know, and I don't care!" was his reply.

I hope you never become so old, or so cynical, or so mentally constipated that you forget how to laugh. Easily and quickly.

We all have to make adjustments to life's joys and disappointments. It is the *kind* of adjustment you make that determines your mental health. Would it surprise you to learn that an alcoholic actually *hates* liquor? Yes, he *hates* it! But he hates the realities of life more.

Impotence can be a form of adjustment. No, a man doesn't just wake up one morning and decide, "I'll be impotent today!" It can be his way of adjusting to a much deeper emotional or mental problem smoldering within him.

The most important thing you can learn in trying to understand human behavior is that no one ever does anything without a reason. The most bizzare or illogical behavior always has a reason behind it.

A man was in the reception room of a psychiatrist's office, stuffing grains of tobacco up his nose. The psychiatrist walked in, noticed what he was doing, and said, "Oh! I see you need my help!" "Yeah," he replied, "You gotta match?"

I can assure you that the man had a reason for acting in such a bizarre way. It is a person's motives or reasons behind their actions that give us the real clues to their mental health.

Thinking of the future rather than dwelling on the past is another sign of a healthy mental attitude.

A man went to a concert. In back of him, two middle-aged men were discussing their operations. "When they removed my gallbladder, they also removed my appendix at the same time!" said one. "When my prostate was operated on, the doctor said I needed a hemorrhoidectomy, too!" replied the other, not to be outdone.

After a lengthy discussion of their operations, the man in front turned to them. "Listen, you guys, I came here to hear a concert, not an organ recital!"

Guilt is an emotion that has ruined many men's sexual functioning. John, a good-looking and successful man, age 53, lost his wife of thirty years to cancer. Since his wife's death he had met a number of women, but whenever he took them to bed he was unable to get an erection. He was examined and there was nothing physically that would keep him from getting an erection. John, however, was suffering, even though no X-ray or laboratory could reveal any abnormality, because the problem was in his mind.

On questioning him, I found that he had an oil painting of his deceased wife hanging over the fireplace in his living room, and every morning he would talk to the painting and tell her that he still loved her. I introduced him to a very intelligent and perceptive widow who seemed to understand his problem. There was an immediate attraction between them. It turned out to be love at first sight and shortly thereafter she moved in with him. John put his dead wife's painting in storage, replacing it with hers. This cured the problem and he was able to achieve an erection without difficulty thereafter.

A young man wrote to *Dear Abby*: "I'm seventeen years old. I stayed out until 3 a.m. last Friday night. My parents objected. Did I do wrong?" She wrote back: "Try to remember!"

Then there are those pathetic cases who refuse to forego their harmful habits and exercise control over their own bodies.

I am reminded of a story told by Benjamin Franklin in his autobiography. When Ben was a young boy, his father gave him a dollar and told him that he could spend it as he wished. Young Franklin went to a corner store where he saw a whistle. The whistle cost a dollar, but he wanted it so badly that he bought it. After blowing it for a short while, he quickly tired of the novelty. Later, his father asked him how he had spent his money.

"I bought a whistle with it, Father," Ben replied.

His father shook his head and remarked, "Son, you paid too much for your whistle."

This childhood incident impressed Franklin greatly, and he remembered its lesson well. Later, whenever he saw someone ruining his life for a few moments of self-indulgence in harmful habits, he would say to himself, "He's paying too much for his whistle."

Then there are the fools who think that money or drugs can solve all their problems, or that they can *buy* health, potency, optimism, wisdom, knowledge and love. Albert Einstein once said, "No wealth in the world can help humanity forward, even in the hands of the most devoted worker in this cause . . . Can anyone imagine Moses, Jesus, or Gandhi armed with the moneybags of Carnegie?"

It reminds me of the parable of a wise man who was sitting on top of a mountain meditating over a jug of water. A villager, observing him, inquired of the sage: "Tell me, what is the secret of your wisdom?"

The learned man replied, "I fast, meditate, and sip this water when I am thirsty." The villager implored him: "Please, I must have some of that water. Name your price!"

Reluctantly the pundit agreed to sell him a pitcherful of water for a piece of gold.

After paying him, the villager eagerly gulped down the water. After a few minutes of reflecting over the transaction, the naive one complained to the savant, "Why did I have to pay for this water when I could have gone directly to the spring and obtained it for nothing?"

"See!" exclaimed the wise one triumphantly, "You're getting smarter already!"

Optimism and laughter can be your best medicine. When an infant never laughs, it is one of the signs of mental retardation. We must learn to be more optimistic and learn healthy adjustments to life's problems. The only people who are *permanently* well-adjusted are in the cemetery!

Norman Cousins, in his book *The Healing Heart*, told how watching comedy movies helped him recover from heart disease. Laughter, he said, was his best medicine.

There was a man suffering from depression. He went to a psychiatrist. The psychiatrist, after examining him, finally said, "Your only trouble is that you have to learn to laugh. Why don't you go down to Radio City Center—they have a comedian down there who's hilarious! You must go to see him—you'll laugh your sides off! He'll cheer you up and you'll get rid of your depression."

"But doctor," he replied, "*I'm* that comedian!"

We all need to make adjustments to life's problems. As I said, it is the *kind* of adjustment you make that determines your mental health. For example, two women both lost their sweethearts. One woman shot herself. The other looked for another sweetheart. A third woman said, "Why should I shoot myself? I'll shoot *him!*"

Do you know the difference between a neurotic and a psychotic? A *neurotic* is a person who is always building castles in the air. A *psychotic* is the one who moves in. And a psychiatrist collects the rent!

One of the signs of a well-adjusted person is optimism. I was once asked to give an example of an optimist. An optimist is a man 85 years old who just got married and starts looking for a new home near a school and playground.

It reminds me of a venerated rabbi, 92 years old, who lived in a small town in New Jersey. He was highly respected in the community and had never missed a meeting of the town council in forty years. Then one day the rabbi just disappeared into thin air. Everybody asked: "What happened to the rabbi?"

Two months later, he walked into the meeting and nonchalantly took his seat. The chairman banged his gavel and stopped the meeting. He said, "Rabbi, where have you been all this time?"

"It's a crazy world we're living in," replied the rabbi. "I was in jail."

"In jail! Why, you wouldn't harm anyone. Why should they put you in jail?"

"Well, I went to New York City to see a show, when a beautiful young girl with a policeman came and pointed her finger at me and said, 'Officer, he did it. He raped me!' To tell you the truth, I was so proud that I pleaded guilty!"

This book is therapy for *me*. I'm in therapy right now! The same principle applies to you, too. When you help others, you are also helping yourself. For example, a tip may be a very small thing *to you*. But it can mean a lot to the person receiving it, whose living depends on your generosity.

You know, stinginess is one of the forms of *mental* constipation. At one time in my practice, I tried an experiment. I let the patient set my fee. When the patient would ask, "How much do I owe you, doctor?" I would say, "I'll leave it up to you. Whatever you think my services are worth to you."

And I found that most people were more generous with me when I put it that way than when I set the fee myself. And they could never say, "You're overcharging me," because they fixed my fee themselves.

Although this system worked very well with most of my patients, there was one exception—those patients badly constipated.

As I said earlier, there is a connection between the mind and the colon. Anyone who lets negative thinking dominate their mind has a constipated colon as well.

It reminds me of a story of a very wealthy but also a very stingy man in church who didn't have his glasses on and put in a ten dollar bill, thinking it was a one, when the collection basket was passed. After they finished passing the basket, he put on his glasses, counted his money, and realized what he had done.

After services, he went back to the usher who collected the money and explained the situation. Would he mind giving him nine dollars change, since he really only intended to put in a one? However, he added, please keep the matter between us.

The usher replied that this was a very unusual request and that he would have to ask a higher authority before he would be permitted to make a refund. So he went to the business manager of the church, then returned and said, "I'm sorry, but it's against church policy to give refunds from the collection basket." The man thought a moment, then said, "Well in that case, will I at least be given credit for the ten dollars?"

Again the usher said, "I'll have to ask higher authority." This time he went to the priest. He returned shortly. "I'm sorry, sir, but the priest says you can only be given credit for one dollar, because your *intention* was to give just one dollar, not ten, and it's intention that counts with the Lord."

You must learn not just to give, but to give with an open heart.

The right mental attitude is most important. Many people still have erroneous mental attitudes, such as, "The world owes me a living", or, "Everyone is against me", or, "Luck is against me", or, "No one understands me". These attitudes must be changed.

Years ago, one of my patients sent me a clipping from the *New York Post* dated September 20, 1972. It was headed "Busy and Boozy Charlie Still Enjoys Life at 130." The article had a picture of a man named Charlie Smith, who claimed to be 130 years old and "did everything wrong." He smoked and drank whiskey "whenever he could get it," and still managed to outlive his three wives.

The article pointed out, however, that Charlie had an easy-going disposition, a quick sense of humor, a smile for everyone, and a desire to keep busy. He worked steadily, picking fruit until he was 113, and then operated a small grocery store. Herein lies the secret of Charlie's longevity. He led a useful and active life. Charlie's positive mental attitude was strong enough to overcome his bad habits.

The optimistic person is usually better mentally adjusted than is the pessimist. He lives each day without mentally dwelling on, "I'm getting older," or his fear of dying.

There is a story of an extreme pessimist who reads obituary columns every morning while still in bed—and if his name isn't on it, he knows he's still alive, so he gets dressed.

There is another story that Miami Beach real estate brokers like to tell to show how long people live there: An eighty-year-old man who lived in Miami Beach wanted to buy an oceanfront property. But the deal fell through because it only had a ninety-nine year lease and the owners refused to give him an option on a renewal! Now *that* man is what I call an optimist!

Chapter 9

Infertility: Causes And Solutions

MAHATMA GANDHI ONCE SAID THAT THE problem with birth control is that the wrong people are using it: those who should, aren't, and those who shouldn't, are. It seems like half the population is trying to get pregnant, while the other half is trying to figure ways to avoid it.

Fifteen percent of American couples are infertile, and desperately desire to have children. Sometimes the answer is simple, sometimes woefully complex. Robert and Martha are typical:

"My wife and I have been trying to have a baby for two years. The doctors can't find any reason why my wife can't get pregnant. My sperm count has been fine on some tests and poor on others. What could be the cause of such variation? Could this be why she can't get pregnant?"

Infertility can be caused by a number of factors besides congenital and hormonal problems. And too often the male side of the equation is overlooked.

For example, human sperm tend to deteriorate and become nonviable at temperatures of the human body (98.6 degrees F. or higher). The Supreme Engineer who designed the human body did not attach the testicles to the body, but suspended them at a distance—so that sperm could be cool, viable and able to procreate.

This is why men whose occupations require sitting for long periods of time, such as office workers, truck and taxi drivers, judges, etc., tend toward lower sperm counts than average.

One case involved Dan and Susan, who tried for years to conceive a child. When Dan's sperm was examined, the count was low, with many non-motile, non-viable sperm.

After questioning him about his lifestyle, the first thing I did was advise Dan to change his underwear from the tight-fitting "jockey" briefs (which they both considered to be "sexy") to the more loose-fitting boxer shorts which allowed more air to circulate and cool off his testicles.

This simple change resulted in Susan conceiving shortly thereafter and giving birth to a beautiful, healthy boy!

Another couple, Gary and Laura, believed Gary had a very low sperm count and therefore was sterile. When they had intercourse, using a special condom instead of having Gary masturbate to obtain the specimen, his sperm count was found to be normal. When taking a semen specimen for a sperm count, a sample from actual sexual intercourse, using a special condom for the purpose, gives a higher sperm count than a specimen from masturbation.

The couple should use a special condom that *doesn't* contain spermicide, such as a milex sheath, or else they should use a well-washed-out condom. Both Vaseline (petroleum jelly) and K-Y jelly are spermicidal. Saliva is a better lubricant.

Can using hot tubs cause infertility?

Recent tests involving five fertile male volunteers who sat in a hot tub heated to 102.4 degrees F. for only one hour resulted in a decline in sperm production and motility, lasting up to six weeks. (*Ob. Gyn. News* 21:12:16, 1986)

Jack and Annette desperately wanted a child of their own, but Annette was unable to conceive. Upon questioning them about their life-style, I discovered that they owned a Jacuzzi that swirled very hot water and the couple had the habit of taking a hot bath together before sexual congress. After I advised them to stop using the hot tub and take a lukewarm or cool shower instead, Annette conceived and shortly thereafter had a healthy baby girl, whom I helped deliver!

Hypothermia as a Treatment for Infertility.

The observation that testis temperature is higher in men with subfertile semen than in normal controls has led to a device that creates hypothermia of the testis in order to improve male fertility. One of the manufacturers of these devices claims a 73% success rate in improving sperm motility and sperm count. This is a new concept which has given rise to new diagnostic and therapeutic technology.

A candidate for hypothermia should have subfertile semen, a high intrascrotal temperature, and a mate judged medically able to conceive. If a patient meets all the criteria, and is fitted for a testicular hypothermia device, it is worn like a suspensory covering the scrotal contents during the time the patient is up and clothed. At night or when in bed, the patient is asked to sleep without clothing over the sex organs.

Research is now going on, using this same principle of heat to immobilize the sperm. It entails immersing the testicles in a basin of hot water for a period of time immediately before sexual congress as a form of male birth control.

One additional word of caution, about hot tubs or hot baths, to pregnant women: *Don't ever take a hot bath or enter a hot tub while you are pregnant!* Hot tubs can do serious damage to the fetus, resulting in birth defects.

According to recent research reported in the *British Medical Journal* (*Lancet* 1:1453, Dec. 24-31, 1988), even two cups of coffee a day may decrease a woman's chances of getting pregnant. According to the report, women who consume no more than one cup of coffee a day have twice the probability of becoming pregnant as do those whose caffeine consumption is higher.

It should be kept in mind that other beverages besides coffee, such as soft drinks and tea, may also contain caffeine.

What are the most common causes of infertility in women?

There can be many causes, but the most common are ovulatory failure or defect, tubal obstructions or adhesions, endometriosis, and uterine myomas. A physician often has to be like a Sherlock Holmes and eliminate the improbable or impossible causes, leaving what is left as probable or possible causes.

For example, a woman who suffers from premenstrual syndrome (PMS) usually ovulates every month so a gynecologist would probably look elsewhere first for the cause. The journey of the ovum through the fallopian tube and finally into the uterus after fertilization is extremely hazardous. Many events must work in precise synchronization in order for successful pregnancy to occur.

Chapter 10

Questions You "Dared Not Ask ..." Answered Here

F OR OVER FIFTEEN YEARS I HAVE BEEN
writing a medical question and answer column for
Nutrition Health Review and *Consumer's Medical Journal*
(both at 171 Madison Avenue, New York, New York 10016).
Many of the following questions were received from readers of
my column. I have included many questions from female
readers since they are the other half of the sex and potency
equation.

I want to emphasize that the information herein supplied
is not meant to be prescriptive. A physician should be consulted
where serious conditions exist.

Arthritic Pain

Q. Is it scientifically true that sexual activity can relieve
arthritic pain?

A. There may be some truth in that assumption. There is
the scientific fact that pleasurable activity can relieve pain. The
brain releases *endorphins*, morphine-like neuropeptides, when
stimulated by vigorous activity. Exercise can also provoke such
phenomena, so can long-distance running. One reason runners

seem to catch a "second wind" and become exhilarated is their reaction to the heavy flow of *endorphins* in the bloodstream. Joggers know the feeling.

Impotence and Atherosclerosis

Q. Is there a link between impotence and atherosclerosis?

A. It is now known that about half the men suffering from impotence have insufficient blood flow into the penile arteries to sustain an erection. Atherosclerosis is *not* a local condition, but is systemic, or found throughout the body. In studies at the Veterans Administration Medical Center in Sepulveda, California, it was found that men with impaired penile blood flow have a significantly greater likelihood of having a myocardial infarction or cerebrovascular accident, compared with men of similar age bracket demonstrating normal penile blood flow.

Men who are impotent and over forty should be evaluated for psychogenic causes and if findings are negative, a vascular study should follow.

Alzheimer's Disease, Affect on Sexuality

Q. Does Alzheimer's disease affect sexual behavior?

A. According to the book, *Dementia: A Clinical Approach*, by J.L. Cummings and D.F. Benson (Boston: Butterworth, 1983), 5% of those over 65 years of age are severely demented and 10% to 15% are mildly or moderately intellectually impaired. Dementia of the Alzheimer type (DAT) is the most common type of dementia in the elderly, averaging about half of all cases.

Although there are few studies on record regarding sexual interest and performance of those suffering from Alzheimer's, the medical journal *Medical Aspects of Human Sexuality* interviewed the wives of 26 male DAT patients and reported: 1) less interest in sex by eight of the DAT patients after onset of the disease; 2) greater libido exhibited by four DAT patients who wanted more frequent sexual activity than before onset of illness; 3) ten of the wives were "unable" to have sexual relations with their husbands even though the husbands wanted sex.

The report also cited hypersexuality in several case studies, such as a Mr. B., a 68-year-old accountant who exhibited progressive memory loss and was asked to retire.

Three years after his first DAT symptoms appeared, Mr. B. "demanded sexual relations four to six times a day, often awakening his sleeping spouse for the purpose of having sex." His approach also had changed. "He was no longer concerned about his wife's feelings, and she reported that he made her feel like a 'sex object' rather than his wife."

His behavior distressed her, and while she didn't want to deny him this aspect of her marital life, she found herself refusing his sexual advances. "In time, Mrs. B. learned to redirect her husband's sexual advances to other activities, and she started to go to bed later after he had fallen asleep. These strategies allowed their relationship to continue less stressfully despite his altered behavior."

Bicycle Riding and Sex Decline

Q. I'm a long-distance bicycle rider. Is it a coincidence that I lose sexual interest for weeks after a trip? Can such activity contribute to sexual decline?

A. It is not the long-distance bicycle riding in itself but the narrow so-called racing seat that can cause the problem. The wide seat distributes the body weight to the ischium or lower portion of the hip bone, whereas the narrow seat puts undue pressure on the penile arteries causing trauma to the sensory nerve that governs erection.

The resultant ischemia, due to obstruction of the circulation, can cause permanent changes in the penile arteries in direct relationship to the perineal trauma.

Narrow bicycle seats should be used for short sprints only, and the wide bicycle seat should be adapted for all other uses.

Blood in Semen (Hematospermia)

Q. I have noticed blood in my semen. I am 28 years old and worried.

A. *Hematospermia* is not uncommon. Patients who notice blood in their semen may develop an anxiety about venereal disease, or feel that they have some kind of sexual dysfunction. But in most patients under thirty this condition is associated with infections or inflammations, and is usually benign.

The patient's precise history is most important to the doctor in evaluating *hematospermia*. In young patients with no history of urologic symptoms, an extensive evaluation will prove no cause for concern.

The condition is usually considered more serious in patients over forty, especially if it is in combination with other urologic symptoms.

Male Breast Enlargement

Q. My son, age 12, has been developing breasts. How serious is this condition?

A. Very rarely is breast enlargement a cause for medical concern. However, it is understandable that it can be cosmetically embarrassing to some men and boys. Sometimes just losing a few pounds can solve the problem for some obese males. It may also be a side effect from some drugs, and rarely, from serious disease. The condition often occurs in alcoholics, since the alcohol can cause testicular atrophy, which curtails testosterone secretion.

If he is a meat-eater, consider the possibility of hormone ingestion. Most animal products contain high levels of the chemical.

Bowenoid Papulosis

Q. My husband has been diagnosed as suffering from *Bowenoid Papulosis*. Can his condition endanger me?

A. *Bowenoid Papulosis* is considered to be a sexually transmitted disease transmitted by the *papillomavirus type 16*. It is most common in sexually active adults, but all age groups are susceptible to the disease.

Bowenoid Papulosis manifests itself as pink, reddish or violet papules, generally flat with a smooth velvet-like surface. In men, the papules are usually located on the shaft and head of the glans penis; in women, they appear on the vulva, labia minor and majora, and adjacent skin; also the perianal area. Women usually experience associated vaginal discharge.

It is important for both partners to be tested for *Bowenoid Papulosis*, and also for cervical carcinoma and cervical dysplasia in the female. A pap smear and colposcopic examination should be performed. The disease is treatable through drugs and/or surgery.

Male Fertility—Vitamin C

Q. Is there any truth to the rumor that Vitamin C aids male fertility?

A. A study by Earl B. Dawson, Ph.D., at the University of Texas, demonstrated that a deficiency of Vitamin C in guinea pigs resulted in 50% loss in fertility within three weeks. In test tube experiments, normal sperm tended to clump together when seminal plasma was low or deficient in ascorbic acid. However, when ascorbic acid was added to the test tube, the sperm normalized.

Another study, announced by the New York Academy of Sciences, involved men between the ages of 21 and 55 who were selected on the basis of the ratio in which their sperm coagulated compared with their overall sperm count. Only those with a coagulation ratio of 25% or greater were selected for the test. Each participant was given either 200 or 1000 mg. of ascorbic acid daily except those in the control group who were given only a placebo.

The seminal fluid of all participants was analyzed weekly for three weeks. Of the men receiving the ascorbic acid, the sperm quality improved in relation to the blood levels of Vitamin C, while the sperm quality of the control group exhibited no improvement.

The important changes noted were increased sperm count motility and viability and decreased sperm coagulation and structural sperm abnormalities.

Candidiasis

Q. My wife has been having bouts of vaginal candidiasis, which keep recurring. She was advised to use the pill or have me use a condom. Since I started using a condom, the infection cleared up, but I am still wondering if the diaphragm is really the culprit.

A. It could be that the spermacide used with the diaphragm caused an imbalance in the bacterial flora, permitting the candida to take over, or there could be an allergy to the chemicals. If the allergen is unknown, sometimes antihistamines may help suppress the symptoms. I would continue using the condom to prevent reinfection.

Contraceptive Sponge and Yeast Infection (Candidiasis)

Q. What is your opinion of the contraceptive sponge? Is it effective? Could it be a source of contamination?

A. The contraceptive sponge containing nonoxynol-9, according to a study conducted in Thailand by Family Health International and published in the *Journal of the American Medical Association* (May 1, 1987) may inhibit a variety of sexually transmitted organisms, including those responsible for gonorrhea, chlamydia, genital herpes, syphilis, trichomoniasis, and Acquired Immune Deficiency Syndrome (AIDS).

One particular disadvantage of the sponge, however, may be an increase in the development of a vaginal yeast infection (candidiasis). The spermicide in the sponge has more antibacterial than antifungal properties causing yeast overgrowth. The more you use the sponge, the more you are likely to develop a yeast infection.

Coffee and Sex

Q. Is it possible that drinking a cup of coffee a day stimulates sexual desire? I am a 60-year-old female.

A. A recent study at William Beaumont Hospital in Royal Oak, Michigan, showed that, of 185 women who drank coffee, 62% reported that they engaged in sexual activity, while only 37.5% of 40 women who did not drink coffee engaged in sexual activity.

Among male coffee drinkers, there was a prevalence of sexual activity among those who drank at least one cup a day. It is believed the coffee raised the blood pressure going to the penile arteries.

Erection Difficulties—Foods which Increase Potency

Q. I am a man 62 years of age, married, and lately have been experiencing difficulty in achieving an erection even once a month. Are there any foods which increase or decrease potency?

A. There are many theories about why some men lose their sexual potency sooner than others. A few people understand the functioning of their sexual apparatus. There are men in good health over 90 years of age, still able to perform sexually.

Let us examine the sexual act physiologically. When a man becomes sexually excited, the brain sends a signal to the nervous system and the entire pelvic area becomes congested with blood. Blood flows into the spongy compartments of the *corpora cavernosa* of the male genital, expanding the tubular rods, making them rigid, while the outlet valves close so that the blood remains imprisoned, causing the penis to become swollen and stiff.

It is simply the blood filling the *corpora cavernosa* that causes *hyperemia* (engorgement), thus promoting an erection. Naturally, all this is dependent on the penile artery supplying blood freely to the *corpora cavernosa*. Should the penile artery become blocked, through cholesterol buildup, an erection cannot be attained or maintained.

There are of course many reasons for impotency, mental as well as physical. However, since vegetarian foods contain no cholesterol, my theory is they will not contribute to a cholesterol buildup in the penile artery and thus reduce or eliminate potency.

Sexual Headaches

Q. I suffer headaches after being intimate. I know it's not psychological. What are the physical possibilities?

A. There are several types of headaches which may result from sexual intercourse. If it just occurs occasionally, it is probably caused by stress or undue exertion. However, during sexual congress the blood pressure rises dramatically in spurts and sometimes, although rarely, may result in a subarachnoid hemorrhage due to rupture of an arterial aneurysm. There are other forms of accidents which may occur to the cerebrovascular system during intercourse which may indicate a need for more investigation, including possible hospitalization.

Headaches

Q. I sometimes suffer headaches after severe exertion (running, moving furniture, etc.). They are not unlike sexual headaches I experience when not in the mood. Is there a link?

A. As there are several possibilities which can be the root cause of these conditions, I suggest that you first have a complete physical exam followed by a cranial tomographic (CT) scan, and a neurological exam. If all of these are normal, I suspect that your exertional headaches, while of a different physiological cause than your sexual headaches, may be triggered by the latter. In the future I suggest that you refrain from further sexual or physical activity until the headache has disappeared. If the headaches persist, I suggest that you consult your physician again.

Hot Tubs and Male Infertility

Q. Can using hot bath tubs cause infertility?

A. Recent tests, involving five fertile male volunteers who sat in a hot tub heated to 102.4 degrees F. for only one hour, resulted in a decline in sperm production and motility lasting up to six weeks.

Causes of Impotence

Q. I have just passed my 60th birthday and find that sex interests me less than ever. Is this abnormal for an otherwise healthy man?

A. Theoretically, a healthy male can retain the ability to perform sexually at any age. There have been cases on record where a man over 90 has even claimed to father a child. I use the word "claimed" since until just recently it has been impossible to establish paternity 100%. However, generally, as a man ages, the frequency and intensity of sexual activity diminishes. For instance, 65% of men between 60 and 70 years of age report sexual interest, while only 20% of those over age 70 express a continued interest in sex.

There are of course many reasons for male impotence which can occur at any age. *Psychogenic causes* are said to be the underlying cause in over 35% of all patients who complain of impotence. If a man has erections during the night or in the morning, the cause of the impotence may well be psychogenic.

Vascular causes are also common because of atherosclerosis of the penile blood vessels. A diet of cholesterol-free or low-cholesterol foods is usually indicated in these cases.

Pharmacologic Causes. Many drugs can produce impotence. Most antipsychotic agents, and many antihypertensive drugs, tranquilizers, antihistamines, antidepressants, alcohol and narcotics may cause impotence. Long-term use of digoxin may lower serum testosterone levels producing penile dysfunction.

Disease. There are numerous diseases that can lead to impotence. Diabetes, spinal cord disease, total prostatectomy, multiple sclerosis, Peyronie's disease, and complications of priapism are some of the most common causes of penile impotence.

Impotence and Tagamet

Q. I am a man in my early fifties and take Tagamet (a brand of cimetidine) for ulcers. Coincidentally, my sexual interest has waned since starting this drug. Is there a connection?

A. Although there have been reports of reversible impotence in patients receiving Tagamet, particularly in high doses, that have appeared in the *New England Journal of Medicine* and other medical journals, Allen Wachter, Manager of Scientific Information, Smith Kline and French Laboratories, manufacturers of Tagamet, states: "Impotence has been reported with Tagamet, but occurs less frequently than in the population at large—that is, people who receive no medicine at all. In controlled long-term studies in patients receiving a single daily bedtime dose, the incidence of impotence did not differ significantly between the Tagamet and placebo groups."

Impotence—Causes

Q. Is impotence inevitable as men age? I'm fifty and wondering what to expect.

A. Just as nobody ever died of "old age," impotence is not an inevitable consequence of "old age."

Impotence almost always has the same root causes in older men as in younger men. Of course, as men get older the frequency of erections gradually decreases, but there are cases on record of men over 100 still able to indulge in sexual intercourse on a regular basis. Many of these claims are of course hard to prove or disprove.

It must be understood that an erection is brought about by blood under pressure being carried by the penile artery to the *corpora cavernosa* and thereby engorging the erectile tissue of the penis. Any blockage of the artery will impede or prevent an erection.

The erection is also a parasympathetic function which may be brought about by tactile or psychogenic stimulation. Any diseases which affect the parasympathetic nervous system can prevent or short-circuit the neurologic stimuli. Alcohol, narcotics, nicotine, antidepressants, antihistamines, antihypertensives and many prescription drugs are known to cause impotence and are believed to be responsible for up to 25% of all cases.

A psychological cause is reportedly responsible in 35% to 95% of all men who complain of erectile dysfunction, but with improved methods of diagnosis these estimates are rapidly declining.

A healthy male can look forward to a lifetime of normal sexual functioning, and for those unable to perform, there are now physical, pharmacological and surgical remedies available.

Genital Itching

Q. What can be the cause of genital itching? My father is 65 and suffers from constant bouts of discomfort.

A. The affected area should be examined by a competent physician. Most cases are not serious, but there is always the possibility of a sexually transmitted disease being present. In such cases, the concern would be finding infectious lesions, such as *herpes* or *condylomata*, another virus that infests the genital area.

The possibility of cancer should also be suspected and biopsies of suggestive lesions performed.

Of course, the lesser dangers, allergy, fungus, and psychological factors must also be considered. Last, but certainly not least, diabetes in varying stages of development must be appraised.

Impotency—Hypertension

Q. My husband is 67 and has hypertension (high blood pressure). Recently he has become impotent. Can this be because of the disease?

A. Contrary to popular opinion, impotence is not caused by a muscle malfunction but rather by blood pressure. High blood pressure in itself will favor having an erection, not hinder it! However, the *medication* to lower the blood pressure may well cause sexual difficulty. Check with your doctor on this. He may change the medication.

Impotence and Decongestants

Q. My fiancé is fifty. He experiences frequent periods of impotence. The only medication he uses is a nasal decongestant. Is there a possible link?

A. There have been published reports of long-term use of decongestants being a risk factor in impotence. Incidentally, nasal congestion may also be attributed to irritants in the diet such as the casein in milk products. If he is able to eliminate nasal congestion, and therefore the need for the drug through changes in diet, and is still experiencing impotency, I would suspect other factors, psychological or physical.

Impotency—Temporary Remedy

Q. Is there an ointment that can be applied to remedy temporary impotence?

A. According to the *Journal of Urology* (141)(3:546, 1989), applying 2 percent nitroglycerin paste to the penile shaft is the latest therapy for erectile dysfunction no matter what the etiology.

In a study involving 26 men with various degrees of impotency, 18 responded to the topical vasodilator with increased blood flow in the deep penile arteries with firmer errections after erotic stimulation. Only one patient showed side effects of headache and hypotension.

It is still unknown what side effects on the sex partners may be caused by vaginal absorption of the drug. This potential side effect may be avoided by use of a condom. **Note:** Nitroglycerin paste is a prescription drug and may only be prescribed by a physician.

Postpartum Loss of Sexual Interest

Q. Is it normal for a young woman to lose sexual interest? It seems to have begun a year after giving birth.

A. What you are going through is not at all unusual. Recent surveys show that more than half of all couples experience a decrease in desire as well as sexual intercourse postpartum compared to before pregnancy. Perhaps this is part of nature's plan to discourage pregnancy at this time in order to "space out" pregnancies and allow the woman's body a chance to recuperate.

Just be patient, and your sexual interest should eventually return to its prior level. Continue to engage in an affectionate relationship with your husband, focusing on tactile stimulation, not necessarily culminating in sexual intercourse. Perhaps a more open communication expressing each other's needs and desires will provide a clue to a deeper understanding of individual needs.

Memory Loss, Confusion After Sex

Q. My wife has been experiencing temporary loss of memory after sexual intercourse. Is this serious?

A. According to a report in the *New England Journal of Medicine* (300:864, 1979), Dr. Richard Mayeux of the Neurological Institute reports on two of his patients, a man, aged 47, and a woman, 64, who both experienced confusion and disorientation shortly after sexual intercourse.

According to the doctor, *transient global amnesia* is believed to result from temporary lack of sufficient blood supply to the posterior cerebral arteries which supply the inferomedial

parts of both temporal lobes. Dr. Mayeux believes the condition only to be temporary and "most patients experience only
a single episode."

Orgasm and Aging

Q. My age is 70. I'm a healthy male, but sometimes
experience difficulty at orgasm. Is this part of the aging process?

A. Age is not the most critical factor involving difficulty at
orgasm. Disturbances which cause difficulty at orgasm may be
symptoms of certain diseases, side effects of taking drugs, and
surgery.

Physical conditions which may cause problems are diabetes, various types of surgery involving the neck of the bladder
(most commonly prostatectomy) and spinal cord damage.
Hypertensive patients on ganglionic blockers (i.e.: guanethidine
sulfate), may suffer retrograde ejaculation.

Other drugs which may cause sexual troubles include
thioridazine, chlorpromazine and chlorprothixene as well as
the benzodiazines. These drugs cause changes in ejaculation
such as decreased semen volume and/or sperm count. The drug
amitryptyline has been reported to completely inhibit ejaculation at orgasm.

Penile Device

Q. What is your opinion about the use of an implanted
penile device in dealing with impotence in a 50-year-old male?

A. In most cases, I believe that implants are unnecessary
and only if everything else fails should they be considered as a
last resort. A penile implant necessitates major surgery, and like
all surgical procedures, it has risks; may result in unplanned,
undesirable effects; and may cause pain and stress.

Impotence is not an incurable disease. It is also often misdiagnosed. For example, an organic cause of impotence can be falsely suggested if anxiety over the testing situation, use of certain medications, smoking, drinking, or even depression can be the underlying cause.

A recent paper by V. Michal and associates found that 85% of men older than age 35—who complained of impotence—suffered from blocked penile arteries that prevented an erection. Clearly, a zero cholesterol, low-fat, high- fiber diet should be the first therapy in these cases. There are many treatment alternatives to penile implants that should be given an opportunity, while the results of surgery are often irreversible.

Peyronie's Disease—Aquasol E

Q. My husband, 50, had a lump inside, halfway up his penis. The urologist thought it was a stone, but after tests and X-rays, he told him he had Peyronie's Disease and gave him 15 I.U. of Aquasol E vitamin to dissolve it. We have never heard of this disease and would 15 I.U. of Vitamin E really dissolve the lump? We daily take a multivitamin, 400 E, 500 mg. C, 25 mg. zinc, B-50 tablets. What should we add and could you give us an answer to our problem?

A. *Peyronie's Disease* is nothing new. It has been around a long time. It was named after the famous French surgeon, Francois de la Peyronie (1678-1747). It is a hardening or thickening of the *corpora cavernosa* of the penis, usually causing a deviation or deflection of the erect penis to the involved side. The cause is said to be unknown.

I believe your doctor is correct in suggesting the 15 I.U. of Aquasol E. Aquasol E is soluble in water. Regular Vitamin E is soluble in oil, not water. If the Aquasol dissolves the lump, please keep me informed.

Pinworms

Q. I'm engaged to a woman who is suffering from a pinworm infestation of the genital tract. Is this a communicable disease?

A. Although pinworms are most frequently found in school-aged children, pinworms have been known to migrate and ascend the genital tract and exit through the fallopian tube to the peritoneum. The disease is transmissible through swallowing the ova of the female pinworm, which deposits its eggs around the rectum of its host.

Prolonged Erections (Priapism)—Phenelzene

Q. I am a very tense person and given to depression. The medication phenelzene is the only drug I take for it. Lately, I've experienced frequent erections of long duration. Is there a connection?

A. Experiencing frequent erections of long duration may very well be connected to the use of phenelzene. Phenelzene, an inhibitor antidepressant, can produce sexual dysfunction and it is the only antidepressant that is known to produce priapism (erection of long duration).

The use of phenelzene may have other side effects: the most serious involve changes of blood pressure, mood swings, dizziness, constipation, drowsiness, gastrointestinal disturbances, and blurred vision.

I suggest you report this undesirable side effect to your physician at once, so he can re-evaluate your condition and prescribe another remedy.

Prostatic Hypertrophy (Enlargement)

Q. I am a man, age 51. My doctor has advised me that my prostate gland is enlarged. I have heard that sexual inactivity can be a cause, but I have also heard that too much can also cause this condition. What is your opinion?

A. There are several causes of enlargement (prostate hypertrophy). Sexual activity would certainly appear to affect the health of the organ because it is involved in the reproductive process. Without a prostate a man cannot father a child. Hypertrophy sometimes develops because of the prostate's inability to function normally.

Any organ will become hypertrophic when it is overworked in an attempt to function better. This enlargement is nature's way of enabling an organ to function more efficiently.

Just as the professional athlete and long distance runner develop "athlete's heart," or heart enlargement, just as the city dweller (where there is less oxygen and more air pollution) develops lung enlargement because of the excess work the lungs must perform and, just as in the person with only one kidney, the remaining kidney enlarges, excessive sexual activity could result in prostate enlargement.

Since the prostate surrounds the urethra, when the prostate enlarges, it tends to restrict or block the flow of urine, further inflaming and producing swelling.

Prostate Cancer

Q. What causes prostate cancer?

A. Several important environmental and epidemiologic studies suggest an increased incidence of prostate cancer in association with certain risk factors.

These factors include: 1) *exposure to automobile exhaust fumes or particular air pollution* (Blaire & Fraumeni, 1978; Kippling & Waterhouse, 1967; Winkelstein & Kantor, 1969; Winkelstein, 1982), and 2) *high fat diet and too much Vitamin C* (Blair & Fraumeni, 1978; Graham et al., 1983; Reddy et al., 1980).

The epidemiologic studies have shown an increased risk for prostate cancer in conjunction with: 1. *An increased number of sexual partners* (Schuman et al., 1977; Steele et al., 1971), 2. *Frequency of sexual intercourse* (Steele et al., 1971), 3. *Use of prostitutes* (Schuman et al., 1977), 4. *Extramarital sexual relationships* (Steele et al., 1971), and 5. *An early age at onset of sexual activity* (Schuman et al., 1977).

Together, these studies link sexual hyperactivity and promiscuity with an increased risk for prostate cancer. In contrast, a study by Ross et al (1981) reported in Catholic priests a slightly higher incidence of prostate cancer than in controls.

Prostate Hypertrophy (Enlargement)

Q. I am male, 52, and have been experiencing frequent urination at night which disturbs my getting a good night's rest. Lately I have been unable to urinate at times and have had to be catheterized. My doctor says I have an enlarged prostate. Are there any alternatives to treating an enlarged prostate besides surgery?

A. Yours is a very common problem among men fifty and older. Unfortunately, in some cases this enlargement, known as benign prostatic hypertrophy (BPH), may cause urinary obstruction. One study reported in the *Journal of Urology* reported that approximately 50% of all sixty-year-old men will be affected by BPH. There are currently 400,000 prostate operations a year in the United States.

I am happy to report that there are two new techniques for dealing with BPH.

1) Balloon dilation of the prostate, referred to as TUDP (transurethral dilation of prostate), involves a catheter with a deflated dilator balloon being inserted into the urethra and, after exact positioning, the dilator balloon is inflated. It is essential that the positioning of the dilator balloon be exact, as wrong positioning could dilate the external sphincter and result in incontinence.

2) Transrectal hyperthermia, first tested in Israel in the late 1970s and now also being used in France, with a reported success rate equal to that achieved by prostate surgery and with a virtual absence of complications. The treatment involves a special applicator to apply focused hyperthermic microwaves to the prostate. The temperature of the prostate tissue is raised to 43 degrees C for one hour and administered twice weekly for four to eight weeks. No anesthesia required.

I would like to add that lack of proper exercise, in the pelvic area especially, is known to be at least part of the cause. Exercise can also be part of the solution.

It is a well-known fact, for example, that pet dogs living in apartment houses and not getting sufficient exercise have a high incidence of prostate trouble, while prostate disease is almost unknown in working dogs, farm dogs, Eskimo dogs, sheep dogs and so on.

"Mushy" Prostate—Prostate Massage

Q. A recent prostate examination indicated that I have a "mushy" prostate. The doctor said I should go in for regular prostate massages. Is there any danger from such constant prodding?

A. A "mushy" prostate usually indicates an infection or inflamed prostate. It does not indicate hyperplasia (enlargement) but may symptomize *acute prostatitis*. In acute cases of prostatitis, prostate massage is contra-indicated. There are several reasons why I am against prostate "massage."

a: *It introduces bacteria and increases the chance of infection of the prostate.*

b: *It irritates an already irritated prostate.*

Instead of prostate massage, I recommend certain exercises. One of the best exercises is to "squeeze the buttocks" or contract the large *gluteus maximus* muscles. This should be done several times a day working up to 50 or 100 repetitions daily.

Another exercise which accomplishes the same as the "massage," but without the disadvantages, is to sit on the floor, resting on hands just behind the back, and bounce on right cheek of buttocks. Then bounce on left cheek.

A hot sitz bath should be taken several times daily and a heating pad applied to the pelvic area may help soothe the inflammation and improve circulation of blood.

The diet should be simple and consist primarily of fresh fruit in season, green salads and vegetables. Avoid coffee, tea, and alcohol.

Priapism—Persistent Erection/Painful Erection

Q. I have been experiencing a strange problem—without feeling sexual excitement, I experience erections that do not subside for long periods of time. Can you explain?

A. What you may have is a "priapism," a condition defined as a persistent erection that is usually unrelated to sexual stimulation. It is often accompanied by swelling and pain. Often priapisms will resolve on their own within several hours.

One of the undesirable long-term results is impotence. It is believed that 72 hours of persistent erection may result in fibrosis of the corporal bodies with subsequent impotence.

Priapism can be caused by, or associated with, various blood disorders, most commonly sickle cell disease, as well as neoplastic diseases such as leukemia.

There are many other factors, both mental and physical, as well as reasons still unknown, which can cause or be associated with this unique urologic condition. It is therefore important to seek prompt medical treatment, usually by a urologist, who is best trained to evaluate and treat the problem.

Bacterial Prostatitis

Q. My husband is being treated for bacterial prostatitis. Is it safe to be intimate with him?

A. The micro-organisms that cause bacterial prostatitis can also result in inflammation of the vagina. Until your husband has a negative culture, sexual intercourse should only be performed with a condom. Additionally, sexual intercourse while the prostate is infected and irritated may further irritate the prostate and delay or prevent recovery.

Sneezing After Sex

Q. I am past sixty, and sexually active. My problem is an embarrassing one. After an encounter (not necessarily the same partner), fits of sneezing possess me. Could this be psychological?

A. The nose is supplied with many blood vessels and its blood supply is regulated by the autonomic nervous system. The same is true, to some degree, of the genital erection and ejaculation mechanisms. Both organs are nourished by the bloodstream. Stimulation that sends blood rushing to the penile artery also directs blood to the nasal zone.

It may be that you are experiencing a mild anaphylactic reaction. This is more common in women and it is generally believed that this is because of an allergy to the male seminal fluid. You may be allergic to a substance or other stimuli in your environment such as dust or fumes.

I don't like to suggest drugs in these cases, as sometimes the "side effects" from the drugs are worse than the disease they are supposed to cure. However, if it continues to bother you, ask your doctor about trying allergy testing or a course of antihistamine treatment.

Nicotine and Potency—Smoking and Sex

Q. Can smoking cigarettes harm my sex life?

A. Suppose the Surgeon General were to order cigarette manufacturers to print on their packages: "Warning: Use of this product can kill your sex life." It would certainly be much more effective in getting people to quit smoking than warning against cancer or a cardiac infarction. Tobacco advertisers portray "macho" type men in cigarette ads to imply that smoking is associated with virility. Just the opposite is true!

Pharmacologically, nicotine acts as a vasoconstrictor. It constricts the arteries and blood vessels supplying blood flow to the *corpora cavernosa* penis, or the two columns of erectile tissue on either side of the male sex organ. Nicotine also lowers testosterone and other hormonal levels in the blood. It increases the concentrations of free fatty acids in the blood, a condition which helps bring about atherosclerosis of the arteries, further restricting blood to the genitals.

Tobacco can also ruin a woman's sex life. There is evidence that smoking can interfere with a woman's orgiastic ability. Nicotine can damage ovaries, causing menstrual and ovulatory abnormalities, and decrease estrogen production. It can also lead to early menopause and other signs of aging such as lessened lubrication in the vagina.

Women who are on the pill and smoke have a far greater risk of dying of cardiovascular disease than non-smokers. For example: in the 30-to-39-year age bracket, of women who take the pill and smoke, the risk of developing a fatal coronary occlusion is ten times greater than in the non-smokers. Nicotine excites the central nervous system at all levels and produces tremors throughout the extremities. If a woman is pregnant, smoking can damage the fetus, resulting in impaired growth and low birth weight.

Sexual Desire and Ability—Injections to Increase

Q. Are there medications or injections available to increase sexual desire in a 65-year-old man?

A. There are many causes for impaired sexual ability as well as desire. At least 50% of the probable cause may be physical, and the rest may be psychogenic. There is no treatment that covers all possible causes. To try to treat a man psychogenically, when the root cause of his problem is clogged penile arteries or nerve damage, is just as foolish as operating on a man who has a psychological problem. Before any treatment is started, the etiology, or cause of the complaint, should first be sought.

A recent case involved a man in his mid-sixties who took oral testosterone to increase his libido and performance. The testosterone was later blamed as an etiological factor in carcinoma of the prostate which later developed. Testosterone, either orally or intramuscularly, should be administered only when there are definite clinical indications for it and only under a physician's supervision.

Sexual Activity After A Cardiac Infarction (Heart Attack)

Q. My husband is recovering from a heart attack. I know he's improving because he is beginning to talk about sex. Is there a danger?

A. Sex is usually not of much concern in the immediate period after suffering a heart attack. Sometimes it is several months before patients think about sex. He may be more concerned about *your* concerns than his own needs. Reassuring him that your love for him transcends a physical act and has risen to a much higher and more meaningful level will help him restore his feelings of security, peace of mind, and confidence in your relationship.

Sexual activity increases the heart rate, raises the blood pressure, and accelerates breathing. If your husband has recovered sufficiently and has a strong desire for sexual relations, then, guided by your doctor's advice, the stress level should be kept low.

It would also be best to have such relations in the morning when he is rested, and before eating anything heavy.

Be alert, however, for the four warning signs: 1) angina, 2) palpitations that last more than 15 minutes after sex, and 3) increased heart rate or blood pressure lasting more than 30 minutes after activity. (Symptoms include dizziness, ringing in the ears, or headache.) Also, extreme fatigue the following day is a warning sign. If he exhibits any of these, avoid any further sexual activity until you consult your physician.

Sex Therapists—Impotence

Q. What do you think of sex therapists, and where can I get help for impotency?

A. Anyone can call himself or herself a sex therapist. Since there may be physical and psychological, as well as moral, factors involved in sex and impotency problems, it is best to start with a complete physical examination because the cause may be difficult to pinpoint.

The physical examination should include case history, blood and urine analysis, and an evaluation of any medication being taken (prescribed or over-the-counter). Low testosterone levels in the blood, arteriosclerosis, alcoholism, blood or nerve disease or damage, high blood pressure, or related diseases that lead to narrowing of the blood vessels (thus restricting the flow of blood to the penile artery) may be responsible or help contribute to male impotency.

If there is no apparent physical basis for impotence, it is time to seek a referral to find a psychogenic cause.

There is an organization, formed in 1983, called *Impotents Anonymous* with chapters in many parts of the United States. Besides help and advice for impotent men, the organization offers support and guidance to their partners. For further information contact: *Impotents Anonymous*, National Headquarters, 5119 Bradley Boulevard, Chevy Chase, Maryland 20815.

Sexual Activity After A Heart Attack (Myocardial Infarction)

Q. What is your advice regarding sexual activity after a heart attack in a 45-year-old man?

A. Changes in sexual functioning after a myocardial infarction are very common. Most patients will be able to resume sexual activity after they have recovered, but many do not because of fear. If they do, it is usually not up to their previous level of activity.

A note of caution: After resumption of sexual intercourse, should there be any chest pain (angina), it should be brought to the attention of your doctor before sexual activity is continued. Your physician is the best advisor with whom to discuss sexual concerns and to relieve worries and anxieties in this situation.

Vaginal Dryness

Q. My wife complains of excessive vaginal dryness. She is 55 years old. Does not use the pill, eats sparingly of sweets. What could be the cause?

A. This is a normal symptom of menopause. It is because of lack of estrogen (female hormone). Have her use K-Y jelly if needed.

Appendices

The Super Potency Diet: How to Eat Your Way Back to Towering Erections

The super potency diet follows the guidelines for preventing arteriosclerosis and its devastating effects on potency and the circulatory system. It consists mostly of a vegetarian diet with fresh, unprocessed foods.

All foods of animal origin tend to clog the arteries with cholesterol, while foods of plant origin tend to keep the arteries open. Meat, fish, poultry, eggs, cheese, milk, and butter all contain varying amounts of cholesterol and have zero fiber content.

Fifty percent of all Americans will die of coronary artery disease unless they change their dietary habits. Anyone who has been eating the typical American diet has clogging of the arteries to some degree.

Keep in mind that the more blood flowing to the corpora cavernosa in the penis, the harder the erection.

It is also important to consume the proper vitamins and trace minerals to heighten your sexual prowess. **Zinc**, for example, is very important for reproductive health. The processing of foods removes zinc and so the typical American diet is zinc-deficient. Oysters, peas, nuts, whole grains, carrots, and sunflower seeds all contain zinc. If you take zinc supplements, do not exceed the recommended dose because toxic reactions are possible.

Manganese is also necessary for the proper development of the reproductive system. Good sources of manganese are nuts, whole-grain breads and cereals, vegetables, and fruit.

According to recent studies, **chromium** helps regulate the level of fats in the blood stream, thereby preventing arterioscerosis. Again, chromium is found in whole-grain cereals, vegetables, and fruit.

Iodine also plays a role in the development of the reproductive system. Dulse, kelp, kombu, wakame, nori and other sea vegetables contain significant iodine levels as well as a wealth of other trace minerals. I recommend that you add sea vegetables to your soups or salads at least twice a week as a source of iodine and other trace minerals. Seafood also contains significant iodine levels. I do not recommend that you use salt in your food as a means of obtaining iodine. You can check multivitamins to see that they contain these essential nutrients.

I have been asked about vitamin supplementation.

Since most people rely on fruits and vegetables that are grown on depleted soils, and are often transported great distances and stored for extended periods of time, the judicious use of vitamin supplementation may be appropriate "insurance" for many people.

There is some controversy or concern as to the adequacy of Vitamin B-12 on a strictly vegan diet. Although most vegan people seem to live long, healthy lives and function very well, I still recommend, because Vitamin B-12 deficiency may be serious, though remote, that all persons following a vegan diet should be sure that they get a reliable source of B-12 at least three times a week. This especially applies to pregnant and/or lactating women, and to growing children.

Reliable sources of Vitamin B-12 may be Vitamin B-12 fortified foods or Vitamin B-12 supplements. If you elect to take the vitamin from a supplement, be sure to read the label to assure yourself that the Vitamin B-12 is derived from pure plant (bacterial) sources instead of slaughter house by-products. Suggested daily amounts for adults are: 3.0 mcg (pregnant or nursing: 4.0 mcg). The body can save B-12 and can store enough in the liver to last three years or more, making it unnecessary to consume it regularly.

Further research on Vitamin B-12 is needed, as there is a great deal that is not clearly understood regarding available sources of Vitamin B-12 for vegans.

I also believe it may be prudent "insurance" to take a multiple vitamin tablet in consultation with a reliable nutritionist, registered dietician, or physician who can advise you regarding optimum dosage.

Keep in mind that certain vitamins such as Vitamins A, D, and B-6, and minerals such as iron can be toxic to the body if taken in excessive amounts. Reading labels carefully and critically is an absolute requirement. For advice and guidance on vitamin supplementation, a physician, skilled nutritionist or registered dietician should be consulted.

Easy Weight Loss for Super Potency

No man who wants to attract women, be super potent, and in vigorous health should be overweight.

With this in mind, several years ago I analyzed my caseload of patients and found that about 20% of them had serious weight problems.

At about the same time, a little old lady in her 80's walked into my office and requested a general physical. During her case history, she informed me that her diet consisted only of baked and boiled potatoes nothing else. The reason she gave for this unusual diet was that about thirty-five years ago she had had severe colitis and was unable to digest anything but potatoes.

Upon completing my examination, I found her to be in excellent health, considering her age. Her mind was also very sharp and alert.

I then examined the nutritional qualities of the potato and found that it is composed of 78% water and has more than twice the protein of human milk. In fact, the protein in potatoes is among the best to be had in vegetables.

The potato is also a nutritional storehouse of minerals, including calcium, iron, and high amounts of phosphorous and potassium. It also has significant amounts of Vitamin A, thiamine, riboflavin, niacin, and ascorbic acid (Vitamin C). It is high in nonirritating bulk and fiber, important in maintaining regularity in those suffering from constipation.

The potato is head and shoulders above advertising-promoted diets and fractionated grains, such as wheat and oat bran. For instance, although oat bran has been scientifically demonstrated to lower serum cholesterol, it has the disadvantage of being a fractionated food that is often too rough on the intestinal tract, resulting in gas, bloating, and some cases of colitis with prolonged use.

On the other hand, potatoes are a whole, natural, nonfractionated food that is also high in water-soluble fiber and bulk, but does not irritate the lining of your intestinal tract.

The average person eating conventional foods carries between one and nine pounds of fecal material inside their intestines. The potato, with its smooth bulk, helps rid accumulated waste from our bodies, and acts as a natural broom in your intestines, sweeping out those toxins.

The potato also has zero cholesterol, so that if you have high blood pressure before you start this program, you should be pleasantly surprised after the first month. Many people find that their blood pressure drops dramatically on this diet, often returning to normal.

You should lose up to a pound a day on this program. However, you should get your doctor's approval before starting any weight control program.

One word of caution. The potato is one vegetable that should not be eaten raw, especially if you eat the skin, as I do. The reason for this is that the potato, particularly any green part of the skin, contains significant amounts of solanin, a poisonous alkaloid characteristic of the nightshade family, of which the potato is a member. However, when you cook the potato, the solanin is rendered harmless. Potatoes should be stored in a dark place, as sunlight activates the solanin.

I am by no means advocating the potato as a steady diet to the exclusion of all other foods, as the little old lady did. You may stay on this diet according to your needs.

For example, if you need to lose thirty pounds or more, you should stay on it for five to seven days of the week until you attain your desired weight. Then you can go on a maintenance program, substituting the baked potato combination program for your regular meals any time you put on a pound or two.

I recommend the potato be eaten boiled or baked. I prefer the boiled potato because baking lowers its water content. Under no circumstances should it be fried.

One of the main benefits of the potato is that it will give you that "full feeling" so you can keep your hunger pangs under control. Best of all, you can eat your fill. A six-ounce potato contains only ninety calories, contrary to its reputation for being fattening. Learn to eat your potato for its own sake, without butter, sour cream, gravy, or mayonnaise dressing.

Remember, just one tablespoon of butter will double the number of calories in a baked potato! Learning to enjoy your food without fattening toppings requires a certain amount of conditioning ourselves to new eating habits.

Don't try to skimp on the potatoes but eat your fill so that you won't be tempted by "forbidden foods."

Here are some wonder-working recipes and menus which will not only help your body cleanse your arteries of plaque and cholesterol, resulting in harder and longer-lasting erections, but will also help to prevent heart disease, constipation, hemorrhoids, varicose veins, and other circulatory diseases.

For those individuals with acute inflammation of the digestive tract such as colitis, or if an ulcerative condition exists, all raw salads should be blended until the condition corrects itself. The blending is best accomplished by placing constituents, finely cut, into a blender. Turn on the motor and push down the ingredients with a celery stalk until liquified.

Menus and Recipes for Lifelong Potency and Health

Breakfast Menu For 15 Days

(Numbers in parentheses denote calories)

1. 10 oz. carrot and celery juice (100); 2 oz. raw peanuts (200)

2. 1 temple orange (80); 2 oz. almonds (200)

3. 1 small canteloupe (100)

4. 1 lb. papaya (110)

5. 1 red delicious apple (90); 1 bosc pear (60); 2 oz. pignola nuts (150)

6. 1/2 lb. black rieber grapes (75);

7. 1 fresh ripe persimmon (70); 1 ripe banana (90)

8. 1/2 lb. fresh emperor grapes (75); 1 yellow delicious apple (90)

9. 1 red delicious apple (90); 1 bartlett pear (60) sprinkled with 2 oz. ground almonds (200)

10. 12 oz. watermelon (50)

11. 2 oz. dates and 1 ripe banana (180)

12. 1 medium size bowl of orange and grapefruit sections (110); 2 oz. cashew nuts (200)

13. 1/2 lb. assorted fresh berries (100); 6 oz. clabbered skim milk (85)

    14. 1/2 lb. assorted grapes, apples and pears
        and 2 oz. almonds (300)

    15. 1 jelly coconut or 1 slice ripe pineapple
        (80)

All fruit and vegetable juices should be freshly made. Avoid canned or bottled juices. A vegetable juicer is an excellent investment for your health.

I recommend you invest in a food scale that weighs by the ounces!

Three times per week include in the breakfast menu any nonsugared cereal fortified with B-12 presently on the market, i.e., Kellogg's Nutrigrain . . . Post Grape-Nuts . . . Kellogg's Shredded Wheat . . . Uncle Sam's (and any others). Moisten with non-fat milk or apple juice.

Lunch and Dinner Menus for One Week

(weight and cholesterol reduction)

Whenever the words "combination salad" appear on the menu, you may use one of the suggested recipes at the end of this chapter as a basic model to learn how to prepare and combine the ingredients. After a while, you may dispense with the recipes and you will be surprised to find that you are able to prepare original and enjoyable salads. Suggested salad dressings are also to be found at the end of this chapter. Salad dressings containing vinegar, salt, or preservatives are injurious to health.

MONDAY

Lunch

Large combination salad; *tofu or lemon juice dressing; navy bean soup; 1 cup cooked millet or 1 cup cooked whole corn meal

Midafternoon snack (if hungry)

Raw carrot and celery stalks, sprinkled with kelp, dulse, or other sea vegetable for organic iodine**

Dinner

Large combination salad; carrot and lentil soup; steamed broccoli and string beans; 2 boiled potatoes

TUESDAY

Lunch

Combination salad; cup black bean soup; 2 or 3 ripe bananas

Midafternoon Snack (if hungry): 3 oz. tofu or 1 small baked potato

Dinner

Combination salad; cup garbanzo soup; steamed cauliflower and brussel sprouts; 2 boiled or baked white or sweet potatoes

  *   Recipes at end of chapter.

  ** Sprinkle dulse, kemp, kombu, wakame or other sea vegetable on salads or soups for trace minerals at least three times a week.

WEDNESDAY

Lunch

Combination salad or 6oz. carrot, celery and beet juice (freshly squeezed to order, not canned); 2 or 3 boiled or baked potatoes

Midafternoon Snack (if hungry): 3 oz. tofu or 1 small baked potato

Dinner

Combination salad; black bean soup; steamed fresh artichokes; Steamed fresh garden squash; 3/4 cup steamed brown rice

THURSDAY

Lunch

Combination salad or 6 oz. celery and tomato puree (freshly made in blender); 1 cup millet (can be bought in health food store)

Midafternoon Snack (if hungry): carrot and celery sticks

Dinner

Combination salad; split-pea soup; steamed fresh spinach; steamed fresh kohlrabi; 2 or 3 boiled or baked potatoes

FRIDAY

Lunch

Combination salad or lima bean soup; 2 baked potatoes or steamed cornmeal

Midafternoon Snack (if hungry): 3 oz. tofu or 1 small baked potato

Dinner

Combination salad; minestrone soup; steamed fresh cabbage; steamed fresh brussel sprouts; 3/4 cup steamed brown rice

SATURDAY

Lunch

Combination salad or 6 oz. tomato and celery juice; 2 boiled or baked potatoes

Midafternoon Snack (if hungry): carrot and celery stalks, sprinkled with kelp, dulse or other sea vegetable for organic iodine

Dinner

Combination salad; minestrone soup; steamed fresh greenbeans; steamed fresh collards; 1 cup steamed millet

SUNDAY

Lunch

Combination salad or navy bean soup; 2 baked or boiled potatoes

Midafternoon Snack (if hungry): 1 golden delicious apple or tossed salad

Dinner

Combination salad or 6 oz. celery and tomato juice (freshly made in juicer); Steamed fresh carrots; steamed fresh beets; 3/4 cup stone ground corn meal (can be bought in health food store)

Salad Dressings

Salad dressings are optional and should be simple and governed by personal taste. You may want to use these suggestions as basic models to prepare your own salad dressings. Where oil is used, it should be cold pressed (obtainable in health food stores) and used sparingly. Remember, it's high in calories (120 calories per tablespoon) so use 1 tablespoon at most per person.

(Numbers in parenthesis denote approximate calories per serving.)

Simple, Quickly Prepared Dressings

Freshly squeezed lemon juice (25); lemon juice and oil with garlic or chopped chives (120); lemon juice, water, vegetable broth powder, chopped chives (35); tofu mixed with a little lemon or lime juice (60); tofu blended with vegetable broth powder and chives (60); low-fat cottage cheese blended with low-fat yoghurt, chives or chopped onion and a dash of lemon juice (125).

Italian Dressing

Lemon or lime juice, Dr. Bronner's or Dr. Bernard Jensen's seasoning (Quick-Sip), basil, oregano, and fresh mushrooms. Blend until smooth. Refrigerate. (35)

Eggplant

Take one large eggplant and slice in half lengthwise. Cook in oven about one hour until soft (when you can put a fork into it easily). Scoop out contents from skin and mix with one tablespoon sesame tahine, (available in health food stores) adding more water to make mixture smooth. Add chopped garlic and lemon juice as desired. Add chopped parsley. Serves 2. (110 per serving)

Healthy Russian Dressing

3 ripe tomatoes; 6 oz. tofu; 2 tablespoons vegetable broth powder (attainable in health food stores); 1/8 cup lemon juice; garlic powder or onion powder to taste.

Place all the above ingredients in blender and push down with celery stalk until blended. Serves 4. (60 per serving)

Japanese Umeboshi Plum Dressing

1 1/2 cup carrots, chopped; 1/4 bermuda onion; 2 cups tofu; 1 tablespoon Dr Jensen's "quick-sip" or vegetable powder; 1 tablespoon curry powder; 15 pitted plums; 2 cups distilled water.

Blended until smooth. Serves 4. (110)

Honey Yoghurt Dressing

1 cup low-fat plain yoghurt; 1 tablespoon honey; 2 tablespoons lemon juice; 2 tablespoons apple juice.

Blend all ingredients or use electric mixer to beat until smooth. Serves 2. (150)

Creamy Garlic Dressing

1/2 cup low-fat yoghurt; 1/2 cup eggless mayonnaise (available in health food stores); 3 cloves garlic, mashed; dash white pepper; parsley flakes or dill weed for color.

Combine all ingredients and mix well. 3 servings. 50 calories per serving.

French Dressing

3 tbs. tomato paste; 3 tbs. water; onion and garlic powder to taste; 1 tsp. honey; juice of one lemon.

Mix tomato paste with water. Add remaining ingredients, stirring well. 3 servings. 30 calories per serving.

Russian Dressing

2/3 cup eggless mayonnaise (available in health food stores); 1/3 cup low-fat yoghurt; 4 tbs. water; 1 tbs. tomato paste.

Combine all ingredients. 5 servings. 50 calories per serving.

Combination Salad Recipes

Righteous Raw Salad

Make a bed of romaine lettuce in a large bowl and place the following on it: chopped raw asparagus tips, string beans, raw cauliflower, raw green peas, parsley, raw squash, raw corn, green and red pepper, celery, and raw spinach. (70)

American Salad

Place in a large bowl two kinds of lettuce (such as romaine, curly, bibb, iceberg), celery, cucumbers, raw spinach, green and red peppers, quartered tomatoes, and parsley or watercress. (70)

Farmer's Salad

Place the following in a bowl: peeled cucumbers sliced thin and halved, 1 cup of bean sprouts, green onions sliced thin, 1/2 cup low-fat plain yoghurt. Mix all the ingredients above. Place 1/2 cup yoghurt on top after the salad is thoroughly combined. (170)

Raw Vegetable Loaf

2 cups grated carrots; 1/2 cup shredded cabbage; 2 cups "Wheatberry Nuggets"; 2 teaspoons minced onions; 2 cups chopped celery; 1 teaspoon curry powder.

Mix all together well, Press into loaf form, turn out on platter when ready to serve. Sprinkle minced parsley along middle. (70)

Andrea's Salad

Take one head romaine lettuce and combine with raw spinach in large bowl (be sure to wash well—spinach often has sand in it!) Add tomatoes, uncooked fresh mushrooms, chopped onions or scallions. (80)

Vegetarian Recipes

Pasta Salad

1 8oz. box tri-colored twists; 1 cup broccoli or cauliflower florets; 1 cup zucchini, diced; 2 tablespoons olive oil; 1 red bell pepper, diced; 1 large onion diced; 2 cloves garlic, mashed; 1 small can small black olives (pitted); juice of 1/2 lemon; 1/4 teaspoon oregano or basil.

Prepare pasta according to package directions. Rinse with cold water and set aside. Sauté onion and garlic until soft. Add red pepper, vegetables, and oregano or basil. Cook a few minutes more until tender. Add to the pasta and add the olives and lemon juice. Chill for a few minutes.

Vegetarian Curry

1 cup brown rice; 1-2/3 cup water; 2 cups stringbeans, 1/2 inch pieces; 1 onion diced; 1 banana (not overripe) 1/2 inch pieces; 1/2 cup raisins; 1/2 cup raw cashews or almonds; 1/4 tablespoon curry powder; 1/4 teaspoon ginger.

Put rice and water in a large saucepan and bring to a boil. Reduce heat to simmer and keep covered. After 20 minutes, add remaining ingredients. Cook for another half hour, until all water is absorbed.

Fruit Salad

Combine any of the following fresh fruits: apples, apricots, bananas, blueberries, canteloupe, cherries, currants, dates, figs, grapes, grapefruit, honeydew, kiwi fruit, lychees, mango, nectarines, oranges, papaya, peaches, pears, persimmon, pineapple, plums, raspberries, strawberries, tangerines, or watermelon.

Sprinkle with chopped or ground pecans, almond, filberts, walnuts, or Brazil nuts; or add fresh mint leaves; or sprinkle with powdered cinnamon or nutmeg.

Bavarian Potato Salad

1 lb. potatoes; 1 onion, diced; 2 cloves garlic; 2 tablespoons cider vinegar; 1 tablespoon olive oil; 1/2 teaspoon prepared mustard; dill weed; dash white pepper.

Boil the potatoes and peel (or scrub well, if using with jackets). Slice into a large bowl and add the remaining ingredients. Cool in refrigerator. Serves 4. 90 calories per serving.

Crudités (raw vegetables)

Instead of a salad, serve any of the following vegetables and fruits with a dip: cherry tomatoes, carrot sticks, celery sticks, black olives, zucchini spears, cauliflower florets, broccoli florets, cucumber spears, yellow squash rings, mushrooms, snow peas, scallions, red or green bell peppers.

Suggested dips: Eggless mayonnaise . . . Salsa sauce . . . Tahini, diluted with water . . . French dressing (see recipe) . . . Russian dressing (see recipe) . . . Creamy garlic dressing (see recipe) . . .

Gumbo

1/2 lb. okra; 1 lb. tomatoes; 1 green pepper; 1 onion, diced; 2 cloves garlic; 1 small can tomato sauce (no salt variety); oil for sautéing.

Wash and trim the okra, tomatoes and pepper and chop finely. Sauté the garlic and onion for about 4-5 minutes in the bottom of a large soup pot. Add the vegetables and cook, covered for another 5 minutes. Add the tomato sauce and a can of water. Cook for another 15 minutes.

Tomato Sauce

1 16 oz. can tomato puree or peeled tomatoes (no salt added); 1 small onion, chopped; 1 bell pepper, seeded and chopped (optional); a few mushrooms, sliced (optional); a few olives, halved (optional); 3 cloves garlic, mashed; 2 tablespoons olive oil; 1/2 teaspoon basil leaves; 1/2 teaspoon oregano.

In a large saucepot, sauté the onion in the olive oil. Add the bell pepper, mushrooms, olives and garlic and cook until tender. Add the tomato puree (or chopped, peeled tomatoes) and cook on low heat for several hours. Add the basil and oregano about 15 minutes before finishing the cooking.

Baked Apples

6 baking apples; 1/2 cup raisins; 1/2 teaspoon cinnamon; 1/4 cup chopped nuts (optional).

Wash and core the apples. Cover the raisins with water in a small saucepan and bring to a boil. Let steep for five minutes. Place the apples in a baking dish and pour the water from the raisins in the baking dish. Stuff the centers of the apples with the raisins (and nuts if using) and sprinkle with cinnamon. Prick the apples with a fork to prevent bursting while baking. Bake for 45 minutes in 350 degree oven. Cool, then refrigerate.

Gazpacho

1 medium can tomato juice (no salt added); 1 large can crushed tomatoes (no salt added); 1 large cucumber, diced; 4 scallions, diced; 3 cloves garlic, minced; juice of 1 lemon or lime; 1 tablespoon olive oil; dash cayenne pepper.

Add all ingredients and chill. Garnish with slivered almonds if desired.

Fresh and Natural Applesauce

4 red or golden delicious apples; juice of 1 lemon.

Peel and core the apples. Add the juice to the apples in a blender and puree.

Muesli

1/2 cup water or skimmed milk; 6 tablespoons oats; 3 teaspoons raw honey; 2 apples, grated; 2 tablespoons raisins (plumped); 3 teaspoons ground nuts (almond or filberts are good); dash of cinnamon (optional).

Soak the oats and raisins in the milk or water overnight. In the morning, add the remaining ingredients and mix thoroughly.

Brown Rice Pudding

1 cup brown rice; 1 cup raisins; 1 cup figs, unsulfured; 1/2 cup chopped dates; 1/2 teaspoon ginger; 1 teaspoon cinnamon.

Cook brown rice according to package directions. Place raisins and figs in a saucepan and cover with water. Bring to a boil over medium heat and let steep for three minutes. Add to the rice, along with dates and spices. Line a colander with cheesecloth and pour the rice/fruit mixture into the cloth. Tie and let drain. Refrigerate for six hours.

Whole Wheat Rolls

1 oz. fresh or 1/2 oz. dried yeast; 1 lb. wholewheat flour; 1 teaspoon raw honey; 1 cup warm water (not boiling).

Combine the yeast, honey and 1/2 cup of the water and let dissolve. Mix in half of the flour and the rest of the water, stir well, then add the remainder of the flour. Do not mix. Leave in a warm place for one hour until the mixture has doubled in size. Mix in the flour on top and knead for a few minutes. Shape into rolls and place well apart (they will double when baked) on a baking sheet. Cover with a damp towel and leave in a warm place for twenty minutes until they have risen. Bake in a 450 degree oven for ten minutes, until golden brown. Cool on a wire rack.

Braised Leeks

6 large leeks; 4 ripe tomatoes; 4 tablespoons olive oil; 2 cloves garlic; juice of half a lemon.

Trim the leeks and wash thoroughly. Heat the oil and garlic in a large stock pot. Add the leeks and chopped tomatoes. Cook over low heat for 30 minutes. Add lemon juice and serve.

Salade Exotique

2 17 oz. cans corn kernels (no salt added); 1 small jar artichoke hearts; 1 can hearts of palm; 1 small avocado, diced; 1 small jar sliced pimento; juice of two lemons; 1/4 cup sunflower oil; 1/4 cup cider vinegar; dash of white pepper.

Open and drain all cans of vegetables. Slice the hearts of palm into 1/4 inch circles. Combine all ingredients and marinate for a few hours.

Celery-Pecan Loaf

3/4 cup chopped pecans; 1 cup diced celery; 1 onion; 1 cup sliced mushrooms; 1 egg white; 1 cup whole wheat bread crumbs; 2 tablespoons vegetable oil; dash white pepper.

Sauté onion, celery and mushrooms until tender. Add remaining ingredients and pour into greased loaf pan. Bake one hour in 350 degree oven.

Ratatouille

2 large zucchini; 2 large eggplants; 3 large tomatoes; 1 large onion; 1 sweet red pepper, seeded; 4 mushrooms; 1 green pepper, seeded; 1 small can corn kernels (sodium-free); 2 cloves garlic; 4 tablespoons olive oil; 1/2 teaspoon oregano; 1/2 teaspoon basil; 2 bay leaves.

Sauté the chopped onion and mashed garlic in the olive oil on low heat. Chop the zucchini, eggplants, and tomatoes in 1/4 inch pieces. Dice the peppers and slice the mushrooms. Add all of the remaining ingredients except the spices and corn and simmer, covered, until soft. Add spices and corn and let sit another five minutes. Serve warm or chilled.

Minestrone

1/2 cup dried garbanzo beans; 1/2 cup pinto beans; 1/2 cup kidney beans; 1/2 cup brown or red lentils; 1 onion, diced; 1 large can tomato sauce (no salt variety) 1/2 cup spinach pasta; 1/2 cup pearl barley; 1/2 cup brown rice, cooked; 2 carrots, diced; 2 sticks celery, diced; broccoli florets or cauliflower or spinach leaves; 1/2 teaspoon oregano; 1/2 teaspoon basil leaves; 2-3 bay leaves.

Soak beans overnight. In the morning, replace the water and bring to a boil. Simmer for one hour, adding more water if necessary to prevent drying out. Add more water before adding grains and cook for an additional 20 minutes. Add the vegetables, tomato sauce, and herbs. Cook until vegetables are soft.

Split-Pea Soup

1 lb. washed green split peas; 1 large onion, diced; 4 large carrots, peeled and chopped; 2 sticks celery, with leaves chopped; 3 cloves garlic; dash cayenne pepper.

Soak peas overnight in an 8 qt pot. Replace the water in the morning and bring to a boil. Simmer for one hour, then add remaining vegetables and spices. Cook until soft.

Vinaigrette Salade

1 cup sliced mushrooms; 1 stick celery; 2 cups cherry tomatoes; 1/2 cup scallions, diced; 1/2 cup bell pepper, chopped; 1 cucumber, peeled and diced; 1/2 teaspoon oregano; 1/2 teaspoon basil; 1/2 teaspoon thyme; 1/4 cup olive oil; 6 tablespoons cider vinegar; juice of 1 lemon.

Mix all ingredients together and marinate in refrigerator for three hours. You may also add: broccoli florets, cauliflower, radishes, carrots, snow peas, string beans, etc.

Artichokes

2 artichokes; juice of 1/2 lemon; 1 tablespoon olive oil; 1/2 teaspoon garlic powder.

Steam artichokes approx. 40 minutes (until leaf pulls out easily). When cool, drizzle with oil, lemon, and garlic powder mixture.

Chinese Bean Sprout Salad

2 cups mung bean sprouts; 1 8 oz. can water chestnuts; 1 8 oz. can bamboo shoots; 1/2 cup sliced mushrooms; 1 stick celery, chopped; 1 cup broccoli florets; 6 scallions, diced; 1/4 cup sweet red pepper, diced; juice of 1 lemon.

Combine all ingredients and marinate in lemon juice.

Pole Beans With Mushrooms

1 lb. pole beans; 1 onion, finely chopped; 1 cup sliced mushrooms; 2 tablespoons sunflower oil.

Sauté onion and mushrooms in oil. Steam pole beans (ends cut off, beans cut in two). Toss the onions/mushroom mixture into the beans. Serve warm.

White Bean Salad

1-1/2 cup dried navy beans; 1 onion; 1 carrot; 1 stick celery, with leaves; 2 tablespoons olive oil; juice of 1 lemon; 2 teaspoons "Mrs. Dash" or other salt-substitute herb mixture.

Soak the beans overnight. In the morning, replace water and add the peeled and chopped vegetables. Bring to a boil, and simmer for two hours, replenishing water when necessary. Remove the vegetables and drain the beans. Toss with oil, lemon juice, and herbs. Refrigerate.

Chinese Dinner

2 cups Mung bean sprouts; 1 8 oz. can water chestnuts (no salt added); 1 8 oz. can bamboo shoots (no salt added); 1 oz. shiitake mushrooms; 1 medium onion, diced; 2 sticks celery, chopped; 1 cup broccoli florets; 1/4 cup sweet red pepper, slivered; 1 cup Gautemalan snow peas; 4 tablespoons safflower oil.

Heat oil over medium flame. Add onion, snow peas, and celery. Sauté for a couple of minutes, then add remaining ingredients. Lower heat and cook until warm. Serve on a bed of brown rice.

Turkish Eggplant

2 large eggplants; 2 large onions; 2 large tomatoes; juice of 1/2 lemon; olive oil; dash white pepper; 1/2 teaspoon cinnamon; 1 clove garlic, crushed; fresh parsley, chopped.

Cut ends off eggplant and place in a pot of boiling water. Cook, covered, for about ten minutes. Drain pot, then cover eggplants with cold water and let soak for another ten minutes. Cut eggplants in half lengthwise and scoop out flesh. Squeeze the lemon juice into the eggplant shells and bake them in a casserole dish for half an hour at 350 degrees. Scald the tomatoes until the skins can be removed. Chop the tomatoes and dice the onions. Sauté the garlic and onion in oil until golden, then add the tomatoes and spices. Continue to stir until most of the liquid has evaporated. Add the chopped eggplant flesh and cook until soft. Add this mixture to the eggplant shells and serve warm, garnished with parsley.

Tzimmes

4 medium sweet potatoes; 1 lb. carrots; 1 cup pitted prunes; 1/2 cup orange juice; 1/4 cup raw honey; 1-1/2 teaspoon cinnamon.

In a small pot, cover prunes with water, then bring to a boil. Let steep for half an hour. In a heavy pot, bring 2 quarts of water to boil and add unpeeled sweet potatoes and carrots. Cook until skins loosen from potatoes and carrots, then drain and peel. Chop the potatoes and carrots, then cook over low heat, adding orange juice, spices, and drained prunes. Serve warm.

Cabbage and Noodles

1 large head white cabbage; 1 package spinach linguine, broken in half; oil for sautéing (about 2 tablespoons); dash white pepper.

Chop the cabbage into bite-size layers. Cook the pasta according to package directions. In a large stock pot, heat the oil, then add the cabbage. Cook, covered until tender (about 20 minutes). Add the pasta and the pepper and mix and heat.

E-Z Lasagna

1 16 oz. package lasagna noodles (whole wheat or artichoke); 1 10 oz. package frozen or chopped spinach; 1 lb. low-fat cottage cheese or ricotta cheese; 16 oz. jar no-salt added tomato sauce (or see recipe); 1 small onion; 1/2 cup sliced mushrooms; 6 tablespoons olive oil; 1 teaspoon oregano; 1 teaspoon basil leaves; few dashes of white pepper.

Defrost spinach in refrigerator (about 5 hours or overnight). Sauté onions and mushrooms in oil. Drain the oil. Mix together the thawed spinach, cheese, spices, onions, and mushrooms. In a large lasagna dish, cover the bottom of the dish with half of the jar of tomato sauce. Place a layer of uncooked lasagna noodles on top. Add half of the spinach mixture, then cover with another layer of noodles. Cover with the remaining tomato sauce. Pour 2/3 cup of water along the edges of the lasagna. Cover the dish loosely with a sheet of aluminum foil and bake for one hour at 350 degrees.

Spanish Rice

1 onion; black olives, pitted and halved; 1 stick celery, chopped; 1/2 bell pepper, chopped; 1-1/4 cup water; 3/4 cup tomato sauce (no salt); 1 cup brown rice; 1/4 teaspoon garlic powder; oil for sautéing.

Sauté onion, celery, and bell pepper. Add the water and tomato sauce. Bring to a boil, then add rice. Stir once, then cover and reduce to simmer. Do not uncover pot until water is dissolved (about 40 minutes). Add olives to cooked rice.

Popcorn

Use a hot air popper (no oil). Season with garlic powder, onion powder, paprika, cayenne, or other spices or drizzle with honey or real maple syrup.

Banana Bread

1 lb. mashed ripe bananas; 1/2 cup chopped pecans or walnuts; 1/2 cup sunflower oil; 1/2 cup raisins; 2/3 cup rolled oats; 1 cup whole wheat flour; 1 teaspoon vanilla extract; 1/2 teaspoon cinnamon powder.

Preheat oven to 350 degrees. Combine all ingredients and mix until moist. Bake in an oiled loaf pan for approximately one half hour until toothpick inserted in center comes out clean. Allow to cool for ten minutes before removing.

Nutty Delight

1/2 cup almond butter (available in health food stores); 1/3 cup raw honey; 1/2 cup sunflower seeds; 1/2 cup chopped walnuts; 1/2 cup sesame seeds.

Blend almond butter with nuts and honey. Roll into a log shape. Roll in the sesame seeds and refrigerate in waxed paper. After six hours, slice with a knife at 1/2 inch intervals.

Tofu-Kebabs

1 lb. tofu, cut into cubes; 1/2 lb. mushrooms; cherry tomatoes; pearl onions; red or green bell pepper; yellow or zucchini squash, cut into cubes; oil for frying; lemon juice.

Marinate the tofu cubes in lemon juice. Heat the oil in a large skillet and fry the cubes until golden brown on all sides. Place the tofu cubes and vegetables on skewers and broil or bake until tender.

No-Bake Peanut Butter Cookies

1 cup peanut butter; 1/2 cup wheat germ; 1/3 cup raw honey; 2 teaspoon sesame seeds.

Combine all ingredients into balls on sheet of waxed paper. Press with fork tines to flatten into criss-cross pattern on top. Refrigerate the cookies.

Gaucamolé

1 avocado, soft to the touch; 1 garlic clove, mashed; 1 tomato, diced; 1/2 onion, finely chopped; juice of 1/2 lemon; 1/4 teaspoon coriander.

Mash avocado. Add all ingredients, mix thoroughly. This is good as a dip on vegetables or crackers.

Mock Paté

1/2 cup whole lentils; 1 cup mushrooms; 1 eggplant; 1/2 medium onion; juice of one lemon; oil for sautéing.

Bring lentils to a boil, then simmer for one hour. Drain and set aside. Cook eggplant in boiling water for approximately 25 minutes (until soft). When cool, remove peel and chop pulp. Mash lentils and add eggplant and lemon juice. Sauté the mushrooms and onion in the oil and add to the eggplant-lentil mixture. Serve with crackers (no salt variety).

Hummus

1-1/2 cups garbanzo beans; 4 tablespoons sesame tahini; 6 tablespoons olive oil; 1/2 teaspoon garlic powder or two cloves; juice of 2 lemons.

Soak garbanzo beans overnight in 4 cups of water. Replace with fresh water in the morning and bring to a boil. If using fresh garlic, add cloves to the water. Simmer, covered, for approximately two hours, until soft. Drain the peas and mash with a fork. Add the tahini, olive oil, garlic powder, and lemon juice. Decorate with a dash of paprika and garnish with olives and parsley.

Sweet Potatoes with Apples and Pineapple

8 sweet potatoes, parboiled; 4 baking apples; 1/4 cup raw honey; 1 cup pineapple chunks, fresh or canned (in its own juice); 1/2 teaspoon cinnamon.

Peel the sweet potatoes and apples and cut into chunks. Add the honey and cinnamon and bake for one half hour at 350 degrees.

Formula to Make "Milk" Without the Cow

Human milk differs from cow's milk in every one of its components. Not only are amounts of nutrients different, but their characteristics and chemical composition are different as well. Cow's milk was obviously designed to meet the nutritional requirements of a calf, not a human. Cow's milk may also contain undesirable components such as pathogenic microbes, cholesterol, and a high butterfat content.

A calf does not have the brain development of a human and its nutritional requirements are different. No amount of modification of cow's milk has been able to render it equal to human milk.

I am often asked by persons who are allergic to milk or who are on a cholesterol-lowering program about making "milk" from a plant source which is easy to prepare at home, from easily-obtained ingredients, and without the undesirable attributes of cow's milk.

Most commercial preparations, usually sold in cans, are fractionated components of soy bean, concocted of chemicals, preservatives, simulated vitamins and commercial sweeteners. This chemical cocktail, which our bodies are required to convert into healthy tissue and blood, is then sold at an exorbitant price several times its cost.

I am giving you my simple formulas for making your own "nut milk" at home.

Almond Milk

1 ounce natural raw almonds

3 to 8 ounces distilled water

1 to 4 pitted dates, or a banana

Put all ingredients into a blender and liquefy.
Strain into a glass.

Sesame Seed Milk

1 ounce hulled natural raw sesame seeds

3 to 8 ounces distilled water

1 to 4 pitted dates, or a banana

Put all ingredients into a blender and liquefy.
Strain into a glass.

The same basic formula may be used to make: Sunflower Seed Milk, Filbert Nut Milk, Pine Nut Milk, Brazil Nut Milk, and Cashew Nut Milk.

Instead of dates or bananas you may use uncooked honey. To cut down on calories, use more distilled water in ratio to the nuts or seeds, and use less sweetener.

Use nut milks sparingly if you want to lose weight. *Do not use nut milks as a sole source of nutrition, or as a baby formula, without first consulting your physician.*

Nut milks require refrigeration, and I do not recommend that they be stored in the refrigerator for long periods of time, since they lose part of their vitamin content through oxidation and may become tainted.

Books

Barry, W. *Making Love: A Man's Guide.* (New York: Signet, 1984).

Belliveau, F. and L. Richter. *Understanding Human Sexual Inadequacy.* (Boston: Little, Brown, 1970).

Brooks, M. *Lifelong Sexual Vigor.* (Garden City, NY: Doubleday, 1981.)

Brauer, A.P. and D.J. *The ESO Ecstasy Program.* (New York: Warner, 1990).

Butler, R. N. and M.I. Lewis. *Love and Sex After 60.* (New York: HarperCollins, 1988).

Cant, G. *Male Trouble.* (New York: Praeger, 1976).

Chang, J. *The Tao of Love and Sex.* (New York: E.P. Dutton, 1977).

Comfort, A. *The Joy of Sex.* (New York: Simon and Schuster, 1972).

Downing, G. *The Massage Book.* (New York: Random House, 1972).

Flatto, E. *Look Younger, Think Clearer.* (Miami: Plymouth Books, 1977).

Encyclopedia of Therapeutic Exercises. (Miami: Plymouth Books, 1973).

Warning: Sex May Be Hazardous to Your Health. (New York: Arco Books, 1975).

Weight, Blood Pressure and Cholesterol Reduction Program. (Miami: Plymouth Books, 1988).

Cleanse Your Arteries and Save Your Life! (Akron, OH: Leader Co., 1987).

Restoration of Health—Nature's Way. (New York: Harcourt Brace Jovanovich, 1965).

Home Birth and Emergency Childbirth. (Miami: Plymouth Books, 1979).

Revitalize Your Body with Nature's Secrets. (New York: Arco, 1973).

Asbestos—The Unseen Peril in Our Environment. (Miami: Plymouth Books, 1983).

The Potato Weight-Loss Program. (Miami: Plymouth Books, 1984).

Conquer Constipation—The Father & Mother of Disease. (Miami: Plymouth Books, 1979).

Friday, N. *Men in Love.* (New York: Dell, 1980).

My Secret Garden. (New York: Pocket Books, 1975).

Gillan, P. and R. *Sex Therapy Today: Sexual Problems and How to Cure Them.* (New York: Grove, 1976).

Goldberg, H. *The Hazards of Being Male.* (New York: Signet, 1976).

Goldstein, I. and L. Rothstein. *The Potent Male.* (Los Angeles: Body Press, 1990).

Haeberle, E.J. *The Sex Atlas.* (Somers, CT: Seabury Service Center, 1978).

Hite, S. *The Hite Report.* (New York: Dell, 1976).

Julty, S. *Male Sexual Performance.* (New York: Grosset and Dunlap, 1975).

Kaplan, H.S. *The Illustrated Manual of Sex Therapy.* (New York: Quadrangle/New York Times, 1975).

The New Sex Therapy. (New York: Quadrangle/New York Times, 1974).

Kaufman, S.A. *Sexual Sabotage.* (New York: Macmillan, 1981).

Levinson, D.J. *The Seasons of a Man's Life.* (New York: Alfred A. Knopf, 1978).

MacKenzie, B. and E., with L. Christie. *It's Not All in Your Head.* (New York: E.P. Dutton, 1988).

Man's Body: An Owner's Manual. (New York: Bantam, 1976).

Masters, W. and V. Johnson. *Human Sexual Inadequacy.* (Boston: Little, Brown, 1970).

Masterson, G. *How to Drive Your Woman Wild in Bed.* (New York: Signet, 1987).

Pietropinto, A. and J. Simenauer. *Beyond the Male Myth.* (New York: New York Times Books, 1977).

Pleck, J.H. and J. Sawyer, eds. *Men and Masculinity.* (Englewood Cliffs, NJ: Prentice Hall, 1974).

Rosenberg, J. *Total Orgasm.* (New York: Random House, 1973).

Schwartz, B. *The One-Hour Orgasm.* (Houston: Breakthru Publications, 1989).

Sexual Fitness. (Alexandria VA: Time-Life Books, 1988).

Stanway, A. *The Art of Sensual Loving.* (New York: Carroll and Graf, 1989).

Slattery, W. *The Erotic Imagination.* (New York: Bantam, 1976).

Taguchi, Y. *Private Parts.* (New York: Doubleday, 1988).

Williams, W. *Rekindling Desire.* (Oakland: New Harbinger, 1988).

Zilbergeld, B. *Male Sexuality.* (New York: Bantam, 1978).

Where to Find a Sex Therapist

Check local hospitals, university medical centers, community mental health centers, psychiatric societies, or senior centers. You can also request local chapter locations from the following:

American Association for Marriage and Family
    Therapy
924 West Ninth Street
Upland, CA 91786

American Association of Sex Educators,
    Counselors, and Therapists
11 Dupont Circle, N.W.
Suite 220
Washington, DC 20036

American Psychological Association
1200 Seventeenth Street, N.W.
Washington, DC 20036

Family Service America
11700 West Lake Park Drive
Milwaukee, WI 53224

Gerontological Society
Social Research, Planning and Practice Section
1411 K Street, N.W. Suite 300
Washington, DC 20005

Masters and Johnson Institute
24 South Kings Highway
St. Louis, MO 63108

National Association for Mental Health
1021 Prince Street
Alexandria, VA 22314

National Institute of Mental Health's Center
    on Aging
9000 Rockville Pike
Bethesda, MD 20892

National Association of Social Workers, Inc.
7981 Eastern Avenue
Silver Spring, MD 20910

Sex Information and Education Council of the
    United States (SIECUS)
32 Washington Place
Room 52
New York University
New York, NY 10003

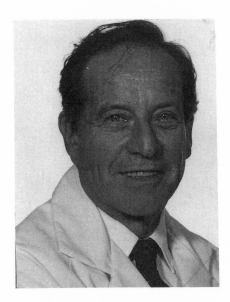

This is the end of the book. But it's really only the beginning for you. Now it's your turn to help yourself. Self-discipline and perseverance are the keys. Remember, I'm with you all the way.

Yours for vigorous health,

Edwin Flatto, M.D.

Index

A

Abkasians, 93-94
aging, 17
    effects on sexual function, 17
    sexual desire and, 17, 222
    sperm production and, 17
    spontaneous erections and, 17
    sexual potency and, 17, 222
Alzheimers disease, 214-215
Antoinette, Marie, 19
aphrodisiacs, 111-115
arteriosclerosis, 31-33
    symptoms of, 32-33
    cholesterol and, 31-32
    high blood pressure, 33
    penile artery and, 34

B

benign prostatic hypertrophy, 37
symptoms of, 37
treatment of, 37-38
The Bible, 12, 19
Bowenoid Papulosis, 217
Breggin, Peter, M.D., 107
Brooks, Marvin, 86
Butler, Robert, M.D., 107

C

candidiasis, 218-219
Carrel, Alexis, 12
Chang, Dr. Stephen T., 155, 162, 176
constipation, 87-99
    laxatives and, 90
    enemas and, 90
    bran and, 91
    foods to avoid and, 95-96
    toilets and chairs, 99
    mental attitude and, 87, 198-201
corpora cavernosa, 9, 220, 224, 237
Cousins, Norman, 198

NOTES

NOTES

NOTES

NOTES